42.95

D1277511

NUTRITION STANDARDS
FOR FOODS IN SCHOOLS

Leading the Way Toward Healthier Youth

Committee on Nutrition Standards for Foods in Schools
Food and Nutrition Board

Virginia A. Stallings and Ann L. Yaktine, *Editors*

INSTITUTE OF MEDICINE
OF THE NATIONAL ACADEMIES

THE NATIONAL ACADEMIES PRESS
Washington, D.C.
www.nap.edu

THE NATIONAL ACADEMIES PRESS   500 Fifth Street, N.W.   Washington, DC 20001

NOTICE: The project that is the subject of this report was approved by the Governing Board of the National Research Council, whose members are drawn from the councils of the National Academy of Sciences, the National Academy of Engineering, and the Institute of Medicine. The members of the committee responsible for the report were chosen for their special competences and with regard for appropriate balance.

This study was supported by grant number H75/CCH324857-01 between the National Academy of Sciences and the Centers for Disease Control and Prevention. Any opinions, findings, conclusions, or recommendations expressed in this publication are those of the authors and do not necessarily reflect the views of the sponsoring agency that provided support for the project.

Library of Congress Cataloging-in-Publication Data

Nutrition standards for foods in schools : leading the way toward healthier youth / Committee on Nutrition Standards for Foods in Schools, Food and Nutrition Board ; Virginia A. Stallings and Ann L. Yaktine, editors.
　　p. ; cm.
Includes bibliographical references and index.
ISBN-13: 978-0-309-10383-1 (hardbound : alk. paper)
ISBN-10: 0-309-10383-5 (hardbound : alk. paper) 1. School children—Nutrition—Government policy—United States. 2. School lunchrooms, cafeterias, etc.—Management—United States. 3. Nutrition policy—United States. I. Stallings, Virginia A. II. Yaktine, Ann L. III. Institute of Medicine (U.S.). Committee on Nutrition Standards for Foods in Schools.
　　LB3479.U6N88 2007
　　371.7′160973—dc22
　　　　　　　　　　　　　　2007023350

Additional copies of this report are available from the National Academies Press, 500 Fifth Street, N.W., Lockbox 285, Washington, DC 20055; (800) 624-6242 or (202) 334-3313 (in the Washington metropolitan area); Internet, http://www.nap.edu.

For more information about the Institute of Medicine, visit the IOM home page at: www.iom.edu.

The serpent has been a symbol of long life, healing, and knowledge among almost all cultures and religions since the beginning of recorded history. The serpent adopted as a logotype by the Institute of Medicine is a relief carving from ancient Greece, now held by the Staatliche Museen in Berlin.

Suggested citation: IOM (Institute of Medicine). 2007. *Nutrition Standards for Foods in Schools: Leading the Way Toward Healthier Youth*. Washington, DC: The National Academies Press.

"Knowing is not enough; we must apply.
Willing is not enough; we must do."
—Goethe

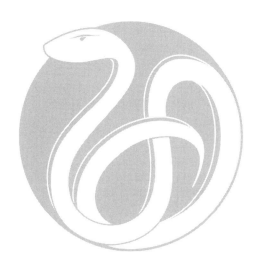

INSTITUTE OF MEDICINE
OF THE NATIONAL ACADEMIES

Advising the Nation. Improving Health.

THE NATIONAL ACADEMIES
Advisers to the Nation on Science, Engineering, and Medicine

The **National Academy of Sciences** is a private, nonprofit, self-perpetuating society of distinguished scholars engaged in scientific and engineering research, dedicated to the furtherance of science and technology and to their use for the general welfare. Upon the authority of the charter granted to it by the Congress in 1863, the Academy has a mandate that requires it to advise the federal government on scientific and technical matters. Dr. Ralph Cicerone is president of the National Academy of Sciences.

The **National Academy of Engineering** was established in 1964, under the charter of the National Academy of Sciences, as a parallel organization of outstanding engineers. It is autonomous in its administration and in the selection of its members, sharing with the National Academy of Sciences the responsibility for advising the federal government. The National Academy of Engineering also sponsors engineering programs aimed at meeting national needs, encourages education and research, and recognizes the superior achievements of engineers. Dr. Charles M. Vest is president of the National Academy of Engineering.

The **Institute of Medicine** was established in 1970 by the National Academy of Sciences to secure the services of eminent members of appropriate professions in the examination of policy matters pertaining to the health of the public. The Institute acts under the responsibility given to the National Academy of Sciences by its congressional charter to be an adviser to the federal government and, upon its own initiative, to identify issues of medical care, research, and education. Dr. Harvey V. Fineberg is president of the Institute of Medicine.

The **National Research Council** was organized by the National Academy of Sciences in 1916 to associate the broad community of science and technology with the Academy's purposes of furthering knowledge and advising the federal government. Functioning in accordance with general policies determined by the Academy, the Council has become the principal operating agency of both the National Academy of Sciences and the National Academy of Engineering in providing services to the government, the public, and the scientific and engineering communities. The Council is administered jointly by both Academies and the Institute of Medicine. Dr. Ralph Cicerone and Dr. Charles M. Vest are chair and vice chair, respectively, of the National Research Council.

www.national-academies.org

Reviewers

This report has been reviewed in draft form by individuals chosen for their diverse perspectives and technical expertise, in accordance with procedures approved by the NRC's Report Review Committee. The purpose of this independent review is to provide candid and critical comments that will assist the institution in making its published report as sound as possible and to ensure that the report meets institutional standards for objectivity, evidence, and responsiveness to the study charge. The review comments and draft manuscript remain confidential to protect the integrity of the deliberative process. We wish to thank the following individuals for their review of this report:

Dorothy R. Caldwell, School Health Consultant, Raleigh, North Carolina
Susan Crockett, General Mills, James Ford Bell Technical Center
Barbara Devaney, Human Services Research, Mathematica Policy Research
Adam Drewnowski, Center for Public Health Nutrition, Professor of Epidemiology and Medicine, University of Washington
Deanna Hoelscher, School of Public Health, University of Texas Health Science Center, Houston
Francine R. Kaufman, The Keck School of Medicine, University of Southern California, Center of Endocrinology, Diabetes and Metabolism, Children's Hospital, Los Angeles
Ronald E. Kleinman, Pediatric Gastroenterology and Nutrition Unit, Massachusetts General Hospital, Boston

Michael I. McBurney, Department of Nutrition and Food Science, Texas Agricultural Experiment Station, Texas Cooperative Extension, Texas A&M University
Theresa A. Nicklas, Baylor College of Medicine
Connie M. Weaver, Department of Foods and Nutrition, Purdue University
Margo G. Wootan, Nutrition Policy, Center for Science in the Public Interest

Although the reviewers listed above have provided many constructive comments and suggestions, they were not asked to endorse the conclusions or recommendations nor did they see the final draft of the report before its release. The review of this report was overseen by **Johanna T. Dwyer,** Tufts University School of Medicine and Tufts–New England Medical Center and **Neal A. Vanselow,** Tulane University, Professor Emeritus. Appointed by the National Research Council and Institute of Medicine, they were responsible for making certain that an independent examination of this report was carried out in accordance with institutional procedures and that all review comments were carefully considered. Responsibility for the final content of this report rests entirely with the authoring committee and the institution.

Preface

My memories of food at school are many, starting with cafeteria lunch provided after we presented our green lunch token and without discussion of choices or options. Everyone had a lunch token, so no one knew that there was a free or reduced-price lunch and no one went off campus for lunch unless you lived in the neighborhood. Bigger or maybe hungrier students got larger portions. A few students brought lunch in cool lunch boxes, and we envied what was assumed to be a better lunch. There were no vending machines until high school, and then the beverages were milk (full-fat chocolate and regular), orange juice, and a few candy and cracker snacks. I think the only soda machine was in the gym lobby.

Hallway or homeroom bake sales provided great homemade cookies, cupcakes, fudge, and brownies. I recall that the school band had the rights to the chocolate bar sale, complete with our school colors and mascot on the label. Birthdays were not celebrated in school. The Halloween carnival was all about food, fun, and homeroom pride for all, from first graders to seniors. Dedicated parents and friends were the band and sport team boosters, and loyally staffed the concession stand for the football and basketball games. I don't remember many students taking time from the action of the game to eat, and we did not want to spend our allowance on food.

This was a time when childhood nutrition issues were iron deficiency and undernutrition, when few were concerned about fat or sugar in childhood diets, and when most meals were consumed at home or school. I now know that some children were hungry and the school lunch was an important source of food. Interestingly, the key stakeholders have not changed—the children, families, school administrators, teachers, nurses, coaches, food service team, and food industry. The local and state school authorities implement federal policy and make many food and health decisions at their levels. In the background, nutritionists, health-care providers, and other child advocates influence both policy and implementation. We now clearly recognize the importance of food and nutrient intake on child health and on lifelong adult health. All stakeholders are concerned about diet quality, emerging food and health habits, and maintaining a pattern of healthy childhood growth. Today overweight children outnumber undernourished children, and yet normal or overweight status does not guarantee food security and a healthful diet for many children. Our inexpensive, abundant food supply, and innovative food industry provide highly palatable foods and beverages for children. School foods and beverages, once almost limited to school lunch, now often include many choices in addition to the federally supported school breakfast and lunch programs. The calories and nutrients consumed at school and school-related activities are an important component of dietary intake of all school-age children. Childhood obesity is often referred to as an epidemic in both the medical and community settings.

It is within this scientific and social environment that our committee established our guiding principles and made recommendations for competitive foods and beverages provided outside of the federally funded school programs. The goal is for schools to employ their unique, long-term relationship with children and their families to support child health and provide a healthful school eating environment. Our committee is a dedicated group of remarkable people from diverse backgrounds and experiences. We quickly recognized that this was not an easy task. Over nearly 2 years, we learned and debated together, and developed this set of food and beverage standards for competitive foods and beverages, if they are offered.

Sincere appreciation is extended to the many individuals and groups who were instrumental in the development of this report. First and foremost, many thanks are due to the committee members, who volunteered countless hours to the research, deliberations, and preparation of the report. Their dedication to this project was outstanding and the basis of our success.

Many individuals volunteered significant time and effort to address and educate our committee members during the workshops and public meetings. Workshop speakers included Richard Black, Karen Cullen, Robert Eadie, Stanley Garnet, Harold Goldstein, Nancy Green, Hope Hale, Mary Kay Harrison, Jay Hirschman, Mary McKenna, Clare Miller, Derek Miller, Alicia Moag-Stahlberg, Susan Neely, John Perkins, Michael Rosenberger, Barbara O. Schneeman, Jonathan Shenkin, Susan Waltman, Shirley Watkins,

Marilyn Wells, Melanie White, Kathy Wiemer, Gail Woodward-Lopez, and Margo Wootan.

In addition, representatives from many entities provided oral testimony to the committee during public meetings that were held on October 26, 2005, December 5, 2005, February 13, 2006, and April 21, 2006. They represented the Action for Healthy Kids, Albert Einstein College of Medicine, American Academy of Pediatrics, American Beverage Association, American Dietetic Association, American Heart Association, Baylor College of Medicine, Boston University, The California Center for Public Health Advocacy, The Centers for Disease Control and Prevention, The Center for Science in the Public Interest, Coca-Cola North America, ConAgra Foods, Inc., The Food and Drug Administration, Food Products Association, General Mills Bell Institute of Health and Nutrition, Grocery Manufacturers Association, International Dairy Foods Association, Irving Independent School District, Kraft Foods Inc., Los Angeles Unified School District, The National Association of State Boards of Education, National Dairy Council, National Medical Association, PepsiCo, The Physician's Committee for Responsible Medicine, School Nutrition Association, Schwan Food Company, The Texas Department of Agriculture, University of California–Berkeley, The United States Department of Agriculture, Westchester Coalition, and the West Virginia Department of Education.

It is apparent that many organizations and individuals from a variety of school and scientific backgrounds provided timely and essential support for this project. Yet we would have never succeeded without the efforts, skills, and grace that were provided in large measure by Janice Okita, Ph.D., R.D. (8/05–7/06) and Ann Yaktine, Ph.D. (7/06–8/07), our Senior Program Officers and Study Directors for this project; Amin Akhlaghi, Research Associate (09/05–10/06); Alice Vorosmarti, M.S.P.H., Research Associate; Heather Del Valle, B.S., B.A., Senior Program Assistant; and Linda Meyers, Ph.D., Food and Nutrition Board Director. Thanks also to Hilary Ray for technical editing.

Last, as chair, I express my sincere appreciation to each member of this committee for their extraordinary commitment to the project and the wonderful opportunity to work with them on this important task for the nutrition and school communities and for the school children whose health and future we were asked to consider.

Virginia A. Stallings, *Chair*
Committee on Nutrition Standards
for Foods in Schools

Contents

Summary

Many changes have been made over the past decades that have an impact on understanding the importance of nutrition in the health and well-being of school-age children and adolescents. Obesity is increasing among this population, putting children at greater risk for other health concerns such as diabetes, hypertension, and cardiovascular disease. Although food choices and eating habits derive from many sources, school environments can have a significant influence on children's diets and play an important role in teaching and modeling appropriate health behaviors.

In addition to providing meals through federally reimbursable school nutrition programs, schools have become venues for "competitive" foods and beverages, those that compete with the traditional school lunch as a nutrition source. These foods and beverages are obtained from a variety of sources including à la carte service in the school cafeteria, school stores and snack bars, and vending machines.

The Child Nutrition and WIC (Women, Infants, and Children) Reauthorization Act of 2004 required each local education agency to develop a wellness policy by 2006. These policies must include nutrition guidelines, nutrition education and physical activity goals, and other school-based activities. Although school districts across the country have taken steps toward meeting these requirements, implementation is inconsistent and in some cases incomplete. In addition, given that each local education agency establishes its own local wellness policy, there is great variety, with policies ranging from very detailed and well-defined, to less detailed and more vague. To augment the local wellness policies and other federally directed initiatives, Congress directed the Centers for Disease Control and Prevention (CDC) to undertake a study with the Institute of Medicine (IOM) to make recommendations about nutrition standards for foods offered in competition with federally reimbursable meals and snacks. An ad hoc committee of the IOM was thus convened and charged to

- draw on literature regarding the availability, nutritional profile, and risks (including substitution) of school foods and beverages, including recent work by the Government Accountability Office, as appropriate;
- synthesize lessons learned from relevant research, development of federal nutrition standards for the National School Lunch and Breakfast Programs, and experience from the development of state- and local-based standards for foods and beverages offered outside federally reimbursable meals and snacks;
- consider whether a single set of nutrition standards is appropriate for elementary, middle, and high schools, or if more than one set is needed;
- develop nutrition standards based on nutritional science for foods and beverages, other than federally reimbursable meals and snacks, offered in school;
- consider how to ensure that foods and beverages offered in schools contribute to an overall healthful eating environment; and
- develop benchmarks to guide future evaluation studies of the application of the standards.

APPROACH TO DEVELOPING NUTRITION STANDARDS

To initiate the study process, the committee developed a set of guiding principles to support the creation of a healthful eating environment for children in U.S. schools and to guide the deliberations and development of standards (Box S-1).

The committee also reviewed pertinent evidence, guided principally by the 2005 *Dietary Guidelines for Americans* (DGA). The DGA provides the most comprehensive science-based advice to promote health and reduce risk for major chronic diseases through diet and physical activity for the U.S. population two years of age and above. Although the scope of the DGA is quite broad, it does not cover all areas of importance to the committee's work on nutrition standards for schools—for example, it lacks recommendations concerning caffeine and nonnutritive sweeteners. However, the DGA are diet-based recommendations, and competitive foods and beverages must be regarded individually. Thus standards were set for individual foods to increase the likelihood that students meet overall DGA recommendations.

BOX S-1
Guiding Principles

The committee recognizes that:

1. The present and future health and well-being of school-age children are profoundly affected by dietary intake and the maintenance of a healthy weight.

2. Schools contribute to current and lifelong health and dietary patterns and are uniquely positioned to model and reinforce healthful eating behaviors in partnership with parents, teachers, and the broader community.

3. Because all foods and beverages available on the school campus represent significant caloric intake, they should be designed to meet nutrition standards.

4. Foods and beverages have health effects beyond those related to vitamins, minerals, and other known individual components.

5. Implementation of nutrition standards for foods and beverages offered in schools will likely require clear policies; technical and financial support; a monitoring, enforcement, and evaluation program; and new food and beverage products.

The committee intends that:

6. The federally reimbursable school nutrition programs will be the primary source of foods and beverages offered at school.

7. All foods and beverages offered on the school campus will contribute to an overall healthful eating environment.

8. Nutrition standards will be established for foods and beverages offered outside the federally reimbursable school nutrition programs.

9. The recommended nutrition standards will be based on the *Dietary Guidelines for Americans*, with consideration given to other relevant science-based resources.

10. The nutrition standards will apply to foods and beverages offered to all school-age children (generally ages 4 through 18 years) with consideration given to the developmental differences between children in elementary, middle, and high schools.

The committee systematically organized foods and beverages offered separately from federally reimbursable school nutrition programs into two tiers according to the extent of their consistency with the DGA. Tier 1 foods and beverages are consistent with "foods to be encouraged" as defined in the DGA. Tier 1 foods and beverages are those that provide at least one serving of fruit, vegetable, whole grain, or nonfat/low-fat dairy. Tier 2 foods and beverages fall short of Tier 1 criteria, but they do not fall outside of the intake recommendations of the DGA for other nutrients such as fat and sodium. Examples of Tier 2 foods include processed foods such as baked potato chips, low-sodium whole wheat crackers, graham crackers, or animal cracker cookies. Foods and beverages that are not consistent with the DGA do not meet the standards defined for Tier 1 and Tier 2 items. The committee developed specific nutrient standards for both Tier 1 and Tier 2 foods and beverages, discussed below. Table S-1 shows Tier 1 and 2 foods and beverages.

RECOMMENDED STANDARDS

The committee's Guiding Principles and the concept of Tier 1 and Tier 2 foods form the basis of its recommendations for nutrition standards for competitive foods offered in schools. These standards have two major objectives: first, to encourage children to consume foods and beverages that are healthful—fruits, vegetables, whole grains, and nonfat or low-fat dairy products—and second, wherever possible in all competitive foods and beverages offered at schools, to limit food components that are either not healthful when consumed at levels exceeding the DGA or fall outside DGA recommendations. Standards that contain specified ranges for fats, energy, added sugars, and sodium are the committee's best judgment based on its interpretation of limited available evidence.

Standards for Nutritive Food Components

Standard 1: Snacks, foods, and beverages meet the following criteria for dietary fat per portion as packaged:

- No more than 35 percent of total calories from fat
- Less than 10 percent of total calories from saturated fats
- Zero trans fat

Americans, including children, consume too much fat, especially saturated fat. Although some fat intake is needed to meet requirements for essential fatty acids and to utilize fat-soluble vitamins, fats are energy dense, and a high fat intake contributes to the high caloric intake of overweight and obese individuals. Consistent evidence shows that diets high in saturated fat are associated with increased risk and higher rates of coronary heart disease. Like saturated fats, trans fats found in hydrogenated oils increase low-density lipoprotein (LDL) cholesterol; trans fats also decrease high-density lipoprotein (HDL) cholesterol.

TABLE S-1 Foods and Beverages That Meet Tier 1 and Tier 2 Standards

Foods	Beverages
Tier 1 for All Students	

Tier 1 foods are fruits, vegetables, whole grains, and related combination products* and nonfat and low-fat dairy that are limited to 200 calories or less per portion as packaged and:
- No more than 35 percent of total calories from fat
- Less than 10 percent of total calories from saturated fats
- Zero trans fat (≤ 0.5 g per serving)
- 35 percent or less of calories from total sugars, except for yogurt with no more than 30 g of total sugars, per 8-oz. portion as packaged
- Sodium content of 200 mg or less per portion as packaged

À la carte entrée items meet fat and sugar limits as listed above and:**
—Are National School Lunch Program (NSLP) menu items
—Have a sodium content of 480 mg or less

*Combination products must contain a total of one or more servings as packaged of fruit, vegetables, or whole-grain products per portion
**200-calorie limit does not apply; items cannot exceed calorie content of comparable NSLP entrée items

Tier 1 beverages are:
- Water without flavoring, additives, or carbonation
- Low-fat* and nonfat milk (in 8 oz. portions):
  —Lactose-free and soy beverages are included
  —Flavored milk with no more than 22 g of total sugars per 8-oz. portion
- 100 percent fruit juice in 4-oz. portion as packaged for elementary/middle school and 8 oz. (two portions) for high school
- Caffeine-free, with the exception of trace amounts of naturally occurring caffeine substances

*1-percent milk fat

Tier 2 for High School Students After School

Tier 2 snack foods are those that do not exceed 200 calories per portion as packaged and:
- No more than 35 percent of total calories from fat
- Less than 10 percent of total calories from saturated fats
- Zero trans fat (≤ 0.5 g per portion)
- 35 percent or less of calories from total sugars
- Sodium content of 200 mg or less per portion as packaged

Tier 2 beverages are:
- Non-caffeinated, non-fortified beverages with less than 5 calories per portion as packaged (with or without nonnutritive sweeteners, carbonation, or flavoring)

Standard 2: Snacks, foods, and beverages provide no more than 35 percent of calories from total sugars per portion as packaged.
Sugars contribute calories without substantial amounts of micronutrients. Limiting foods high in added sugars is recommended because high levels of added sugars are associated with increased calorie and decreased micronutrient consumption. Decreases in micronutrient intake are greatest when added sugars exceed 25 percent of the total caloric intake. However, the committee decided that a 35 percent limit on total sugars (for non-dairy products) would be achievable while contributing to improvement in the eating patterns of school-age children.

Recent data show that added sugars from soft drinks, fruitades, and other sweetened fruit drinks contribute from 35 to more than 50 percent of the total intake of added sugars in children's diets. Decreases in allowable added sugars are intended to provide an incentive for food manufacturers to develop an array of acceptable products that contain less than 35 percent of calories from total sugars. Many food products already in the marketplace approach this limit, and through modest reformulation will conform to the committee's recommendation. With the exceptions noted, the recommendation of 35 percent of calories from total sugars is viewed by the committee as an interim recommendation until added sugars information is more readily available to school foodservice operators.

Exceptions to the standard are

- 100 percent fruits and fruit juices in all forms without added sugars;
- 100 percent vegetables and vegetable juices without added sugars; and
- unflavored nonfat and low-fat milk and yogurt. Flavored nonfat and low-fat milk can contain no more than 22 grams of total sugars per 8-ounce portion, and flavored nonfat and low-fat yogurt can contain no more than 30 grams of total sugars per 8-ounce serving.

Dairy product exception Dietary intake of calcium-rich foods and beverages is very important throughout the school years, but many of the dairy products popular among school-age children that can make a positive contribution contain added sugars in excess of the recommended limit set by the committee. To avoid elimination of these dairy products due to sugar content, the committee made an exception to the recommended limit on added sugars.

In setting the proposed higher standards for these foods and beverages, the committee sets limits that are both attainable and maintain product palatability, while still reducing intake of added sugars. In making the recommendations, the committee is also mindful of the positive efforts of some states and school districts, sometimes working together with the dairy industry, to successfully develop products lower in added sugars.

Standard 3: Snack items are 200 calories or less per portion as packaged and à la carte entrée items do not exceed calorie limits on comparable National School Lunch Program (NSLP) items.
Entrée items served à la carte are exempt from the 200-calorie limit; their caloric content does not exceed that of comparable NSLP entrée items.

Most U.S. children consume at least one snack per day, and children consume nearly one quarter of their dietary energy intake as snacks. Energy intake should be commensurate with energy expenditure in order to achieve energy balance in adults and avoid overweight and obesity; only a small positive energy balance is required for growth in school-age children. The energy density of foods is higher for snacks compared to meals, and excess weight gain may develop over time from a relatively small daily excess of calories consumed.

The committee determined that discretionary energy consumption from snacks should represent no more than about 9 percent of total daily energy intake. A 200-calorie maximum limit per portion for snacks may be high for some younger or smaller children, but it is assumed that variations in other daily energy intake will compensate for shortfalls or excesses. Furthermore, à la carte entrée items should not provide more calories than the comparable NSLP entrée items they replace. The standard is established for whole servings rather than half servings because, in the committee's judgment, a whole serving of fruit, vegetable, or whole grain per portion would contribute to the goal of helping school-age children meet DGA recommendations in a portion size that food manufacturers can achieve in formulating new products.

Standard 4: Snack items meet a sodium content limit of 200 mg or less per portion as packaged or 480 mg or less per entrée portion as served à la carte.
Although sodium is an essential dietary mineral, it is widely overconsumed. Research evidence in adult subjects strongly supports a correlation between higher salt intake and increased blood pressure, although associations in children and adolescents are not as well documented.

The exception to the sodium recommendation for federally reimbursable school meal entrée items purchased à la carte reflects the fact that they generally represent greater energy value than the recommended limit for snacks (Standard 3 above). These entrée items are components of meals that meet U.S. Department of Agriculture school meal nutrition standards and their inclusion allows greater flexibility for students with higher energy needs.

Standards for Nonnutritive Food Components

Standard 5: Beverages containing nonnutritive sweeteners are only allowed in high schools after the end of the school day.
In considering nonnutritive sweeteners in competitive foods and beverages for school-age children, four related issues were evaluated: safety; displacement effect on intake of other foods and beverages to be encouraged (fruits, vegetables, whole grains, and nonfat or low-fat dairy products); efficacy for maintenance of healthy weight; and the role of choice and necessity.

Safety The Food and Drug Administration (FDA) sets safety standards for food additives, including nonnutritive sweeteners. Those that are approved for use have been evaluated extensively and have met the standards. Yet there is still uncertainty, particularly about long-term use and about low-level exposure effects on the health and development of children.

Displacement Nonnutritive-sweetened beverages may be chosen instead of nutrient-dense beverages. Nutrient displacement occurs when a beverage or food of lesser nutritional value is substituted for one of greater nutritional value, resulting in reduced intake of nutrients.

Efficacy The DGA states that reduction of calorie intake is important in weight control. Nonnutritive sweeteners are used to replace sugars in foods and beverages and provide lower calorie choices to consumers.

Choice and necessity Beverages that meet Tier 2 standards make no caloric contribution and increase the variety of choices. These additional choices may be useful for those who wish to control or maintain body weight. The use of nonnutritive sweeteners to provide lower calorie foods and beverages, however, is not necessary to achieve the goal of weight control.
The committee considered these issues in the context of development in school age children and the public health concern of childhood obesity. Given the lack of clear evidence to evaluate their efficacy in weight control, intending to maintain clarity and avoiding complexity of standards across age groups and times of day, the committee took a cautious approach in its recommendations for the use of nonnutritive sweeteners in competitive foods and beverages.

Because of the uncertainties and limitations in evidence, especially concerning the safety and benefits for weight control, the committee does not recommend a standard for nonnutritive sweeteners in foods.

Safety Nonnutritive sweeteners meet the safety standards set by the FDA; however, there is no long-term evidence addressing their safety when consumption begins in early childhood, and in relation to a broader range of health and developmental outcomes. The committee also considered the limitations in testing and lack of evidence concerning the benefits or necessity for use of nonnutritive sweeteners in foods.

Displacement Displacement was not an important issue for nonnutritive sweeteners in foods that otherwise met the recommended standards.

Efficacy Based on the principle of energy balance, nonnutritive sweeteners in foods might provide a tool for weight management; however, studies to test this in children are not conclusive and the complexities of the relationship between nonnutritive sweeteners and appetite have not been studied in this age group.

Choice and necessity Although nonnutritive sweeteners may increase palatability, thereby increasing consumption of healthful foods, the potential increase in consumption may not be sufficient justification to include them in foods. There was also concern that children may not be able to distinguish between a food with nonnutritive sweeteners and a similar full-calorie food, which might encourage unintentional overconsumption. Improving dietary patterns and maintaining healthy weight in children does not require foods with nonnutritive sweeteners.

Standard 6: Foods and beverages are caffeine-free, with the exception of trace amounts of naturally occurring caffeine-related substances.
The evidence for adverse health effects, other than physical dependency and withdrawal, from caffeine consumption varies in severity of effects and consistency of results among studies (see discussion in Chapter 2) except for the two health effects mentioned. Tolerance and dependence on caffeine have been identified in all ages, including school-age children, and withdrawal from regular caffeine intake is followed by generally mild effects such as moodiness, headache, and shakiness.

Although there may be some benefits associated with caffeine consumption (see Chapter 2), the committee did not support offering products containing significant amounts of caffeine for school-age children because of the potential for adverse effects, including physical dependency and withdrawal (described in Chapter 2). Thus the committee judged that caffeine in significant quantities has no place in foods and beverages offered in schools. The committee recognized that some foods and beverages contain trace amounts of naturally occurring caffeine and related substances and did not intend to exclude such foods or beverages if the amounts of caffeine consumed are small and the product otherwise complies with the recommended nutritional standards.

Standards for the School Day

Standard 7: Foods and beverages offered during the school day are limited to those in Tier 1.
Because of their nutritional attributes, consumption of Tier 1 foods and beverages is to be encouraged. Thus it is appropriate to make them available as competitive foods during the school day. Evidence supports the use of Tier 1 foods and beverages to increase consumption of fruits, vegetables, whole grains, and nonfat and low-fat dairy products by school-age children, and to reinforce innovation by industry to create products more consistent with the DGA, thereby increasing healthful competitive food choices for school-age children.

Standard 8: Plain, potable water is available throughout the school day at no cost to students.
Water is essential to health, and is naturally calorie free with few known negative health consequences. Either tap or bottled water or water from fountains or other sources represents a safe, desirable way of maintaining hydration during the school day, and is therefore included as a Tier 1 beverage. The committee's interpretation of limited available evidence is that carbonated water, fortified water, flavored water, and similar products are excluded because such products are associated with displacement of more healthful beverages (see Chapter 2); they are unnecessary for hydration purposes; and the increasing variety of products increases the difficulty of making clear distinctions among them. In addition, if flavored or fortified waters are included, they may serve, in the committee's judgment, as implicit encouragement to produce more foods with nonnutritive components for children at the expense of more healthful foods.

Standard 9: Sports drinks are not available in the school setting except when provided by the school for student athletes participating in sport programs involving vigorous activity of more than one hour's duration.
The committee concluded that, in most contexts, sports drinks are equivalent to flavored water, and because of their high sugar content it is appropriate that they be excluded from both Tier 1 and 2 beverages. However, for students engaged in prolonged, vigorous activities on hot days, evi-

dence suggests sports drinks are useful for facilitating hydration, providing energy, and replacing electrolytes. The committee's recommended standard is consistent with conclusions of expert panels who considered this issue in adults. The committee suggests that the individual athletic coach determine whether sports drinks are made available to student athletes under allowable conditions to maintain hydration.

Standard 10: Foods and beverages are not used as rewards or discipline for academic performance or behavior.
Some schools have reported the use of foods and beverages as an aid in managing behavior. In the committee's judgment, such use of foods and beverages in schools is inappropriate. Establishing an emotional connection between food and acomplishment encourages poor eating habits, and in the committee's judgment should not be allowed.

Standard 11: Minimize marketing of Tier 2 snacks, foods, and beverages in the high school setting by

• locating Tier 2 food and beverage distribution in low student traffic areas; and
• ensuring that the exteriors of vending machines do not depict commercial products or logos or suggest that consumption of vended items conveys a health or social benefit.

The presence in some high schools of vending machines or other mechanisms to market Tier 2 snacks, foods, and beverages after school leaves open an opportunity to promote products during the regular school day, even if these vending machines operate only after the end of the regular school day. In making this recommendation, the committee concurs with the recommendations of the recent IOM report on food and beverage marketing to children.

Standards for the After-School Setting

Standard 12: Tier 1 snack items are allowed after school for student activities for elementary and middle schools. Tier 1 and Tier 2 snacks are allowed after school for high school.
The committee's recommended standard applies specifically to after-school activities that are attended mainly by students and thus represent an extension of the regular school day.
Many school-related activities that take place in the late afternoon and evening involve both students and adults or, in some instances, mainly adults. These include interscholastic sporting events, back-to-school nights,

parent-teacher association meetings, and use of the school for adult activities such as adult athletic leagues.

Some students remain on the campus and proceed directly to their after-school activities, while others leave campus and return for these activities. Some food consumed during the after-school period is provided by the school, while in other cases it is provided by students or others.

Given that high school students are often expected to decide what to eat, it is appropriate to give them more choice in the less formal environment after the school day ends. Tier 2 foods and beverages provide for an expanded variety while maintaining nutritional standards.

Standard 13: For on-campus fund-raising activities during the school day, Tier 1 foods and beverages are allowed for elementary middle, and high schools. Tier 2 foods and beverages are allowed for high schools after school. For evening and community activities that include adults, Tier 1 and 2 foods and beverages are encouraged.

Fund-raising or evening and community activities that include the use of foods and beverages should emphasize nutritious choices such as fruits or juices, vegetables, nuts, grain products, and nonfat or low-fat dairy products. The committee recognizes that attempting to regulate foods and beverages sold for fund-raising or offered at evening events attended by both students and adults is not practical and may not be desirable. The committee urges that when foods and beverages are used for such activities they be limited to items that meet Tier 1 and Tier 2 standards.

IMPLEMENTING THE RECOMMENDED STANDARDS

The recommended nutrition standards are among several elements of a school policy that could significantly improve the nutritional quality of foods offered in schools. While proposing a complete implementation and evaluation plan is beyond the scope of the study, the committee developed a framework and set of benchmarks on which such a plan can be developed. The key elements for success in implementing standards for competitive foods in schools are summarized in Box S-2, and recommended actions follow.

Action 1: Appropriate policy-making bodies ensure that recommendations are fully adopted by providing

- regulatory guidance to federal, state, and local authorities;
- designated responsibility for overall coordination and oversight to federal, state, and local authorities; and

---

BOX S-2
Key Elements for Success

1. Awareness and understanding of the standards by personnel in schools, school boards, school district administrators, parents, students, health professionals and child advocates, state agencies, state boards of education and legislatures, Congress, the U.S. Department of Agriculture, the U.S. Department of Health and Human Services, the U.S. Department of Education, food and beverage industry, and vendors.

2. Actions taken to implement nutrition standards by those same personnel, potentially including
   - Supportive legislation at federal,state, and/or local levels
   - Supportive regulations issued by federal, state, and/or local agencies
   - Technical and financial support as needed
   - Incorporation of standards into school wellness policies
   - Development of food and beverage products that meet standards

3. Changes in food availability in schools, including
   - Products offered in à la carte, in vending machines, stores, and snack bars consistent with the standards
   - Products used in celebrations, fundraising, and after-school activities consistent with the standards.

4. Changes in children's food and beverage sources and intake during the extended school day, including
   - Improved product profile (e.g., servings of food groups, types of beverages, etc.)
   - Improved nutrient composition of children's diets

- performance-based guidelines and technical and financial support to schools or school districts, as needed.

Implementing the recommended nutrition standards for competitive foods and beverages offered in schools will require policy changes. These changes may occur at multiple levels, such as local, state, and/or national levels, and may combine policy guidance, regulations, and/or legislative action. In order for the recommended standards to be implemented, an authoritative agency must be designated to coordinate and monitor progress.

Action 2: Appropriate federal agencies engage with the food industry to

- establish a user-friendly identification system for Tier 1 and 2 snacks, foods, and beverages that meet the standards per portion as packaged

• provide specific guidance for whole-grain products and combination products that contain fruits, vegetables, and whole grains

Implementing the standards recommended in this report for Tier 1 and 2 snacks, foods, and beverages will only be accomplished with coordination and cooperation among federal agencies and the food industry. Product information currently available to foodservice operators is not always sufficient to determine whether products meet nutrition standards. In order for school foodservice operators to identify and evaluate foods and beverages that meet specified standards, detailed product information must be provided by manufacturers.

CONCLUDING REMARKS

The federally reimbursable school nutrition programs are traditionally an important means to ensure that students have access to fruits, vegetables, whole-grain-based foods, and nonfat and low-fat dairy products during the school day. These programs are the main source of nutrition provided at school. However, there are increasing opportunities for students to select competitive snacks, foods, and beverages through à la carte services, vending machines, school stores, snack bars, concession stands, classroom or school celebrations, achievement rewards, after-school programs, and other venues. Schools are encouraged to limit these opportunities. When such opportunities arise, they should be used to encourage greater consumption of fruits, vegetables, whole grains, and nonfat or low-fat dairy products. The recommendations in this report are intended to ensure that competitive foods and beverages offered in schools are consistent with the DGA and, in particular, to encourage children and adolescents to develop healthful lifelong eating patterns.

1

Committee Task and Guiding Principles

BACKGROUND

The dietary practices of children and adolescents are critical to their overall health and well-being. Unfortunately, children's diets tend to be inadequate in fruits, vegetables, whole grains, and calcium-rich foods and too high in sodium, saturated fat, and added sugar. The School Nutrition Dietary Assessment Study II (SNDA-II) (Fox et al., 2001) reports that intake of total fat among school-age children makes up approximately 33–35 percent of caloric intake (upper limit of recommended level), and saturated fat intake is approximately 12 percent of total caloric intake (exceeding recommended levels). Although obesity increases health problems among U.S. school-age children and adolescents, the resulting greater risk that these health problems pose for other serious chronic conditions—including diabetes, cardiovascular disease, and elevated cholesterol and blood pressure levels—cannot be overlooked. Other nutrition and health issues that have an impact on children and adolescents include poor bone health, dental caries, and low iron intake. In addition to these issues of physical health, sociocultural issues are of concern, particularly the social discrimination against obese children and adolescents.

Food choices and eating habits are learned from many sources. However, the school environment plays a significant role in teaching and modeling eating and health behaviors. For many children, foods consumed at school provide a major portion of their daily nutrient intake. Foods and beverages consumed at school come from three major sources: (1) federally able school nutrition programs that include the National School Lunch Program (NSLP), the School Breakfast Program (SBP), and after-school snacks; (2) food and beverage sources that include items sold or offered through à la carte lines, snack bars, student stores, vending machines, or school activities such as special fundraisers, achievement rewards, classroom parties, school celebrations, classroom snacks, and school meetings; and (3) foods brought from home ("brown bag" lunches).

Foods and beverages sold at school outside of the NSLP or SBP are referred to as "competitive foods" because they compete with the traditional school meals as a nutrition source (see Chapter 3 for detailed discussion). Such foods and beverages may include carbonated sodas, fruit-flavored drinks of low fruit content, snack foods high in added sugar or salt, and baked goods high in fat as well as healthier options such as small whole-grain bagels and fruit. A number of factors influence the decision to allow competitive foods in the school environment, including state and local policies, student preferences, commercial marketing strategies in the school, administrative and parental opinions, financial concerns, and time and space constraints affecting meal service in the school. Lunches brought from home are not included as they fall outside the scope of the report.

There are important concerns about the contribution of nutrients and total calories from competitive foods to the daily diets of school-age children and adolescents. First, competitive foods tend to be calorie-dense rather than nutrient-dense and thus may contribute to the increasing problem of overweight and obesity among school-age children and adolescents (Kubik et al., 2003, 2005; Templeton et al., 2005). They may also contribute to other health conditions, including dental caries, poor bone health, and iron-deficiency anemia (Lytle and Kubik, 2003). Second, in contrast to meals served through the NSLP—which are generally consistent with national nutrition policy as delineated in the *Dietary Guidelines for Americans* (DGA)—competitive foods do not follow any federal nutrition guidelines and are not likely to conform to nutrient intake recommendations. Table 1-1 summarizes the recommendations from the DGA (DHHS/USDA, 2005). Third, these foods are increasingly available and consumed in a variety of venues across the school campus and throughout the school day. Given that children's diets tend not to meet the DGA, and there is an abundance of often unhealthy food and beverage choices available at school, developing nutrient standards for individual products available outside the federally reimbursable school nutrition programs will make an important contribution toward improving the healthfulness of children's diets.

The public recognition of and attention to these issues has resulted in a call for effective solutions. In June 2004, Congress passed Section 204 of Public Law 108–265 of the Child Nutrition and WIC (Women, Infants, and Children) Reauthorization Act that required local education agencies to

TABLE 1-1 Key Recommendations for the General Population from the *Dietary Guidelines for Americans 2005*

Focus Area	Key Recommendation
Adequate nutrients within calorie needs	• Consume a variety of nutrient-dense foods and beverages within and among the basic food groups while choosing foods that limit the intake of saturated and trans fats, cholesterol, added sugars, salt, and alcohol. • Meet recommended intakes within energy needs by adopting a balanced eating pattern, such as the U.S. Department of Agriculture (USDA) Food Guide or the Dietary Approaches to Stop Hypertension (DASH) Eating Plan.
Weight management	• To maintain body weight in a healthy range, balance calories from foods and beverages with calories expended. • To prevent gradual weight gain over time, make small decreases in food and beverage calories and increase physical activity.
Physical activity	• Engage in regular physical activity and reduce sedentary activities to promote health, psychological well-being, and a healthy body weight. —To reduce the risk of chronic disease in adulthood, engage in at least 30 minutes of moderate-intensity physical activity, above usual activity, at work or home on most days of the week. —For most people, greater health benefits can be obtained by engaging in physical activity of more vigorous intensity or longer duration. —To help manage body weight and prevent gradual, unhealthy body weight gain in adulthood, engage in approximately 60 minutes of moderate- to vigorous-intensity activity on most days of the week while not exceeding caloric intake requirements. —To sustain weight loss in adulthood, participate in at least 60 to 90 minutes of daily moderate-intensity physical activity while not exceeding caloric intake requirements. Some people may need to consult with a health-care provider before participating in this level of activity. • Achieve physical fitness by including cardiovascular conditioning, stretching exercises for flexibility, and resistance exercises or calisthenics for muscle strength and endurance.
Food groups to encourage	• Consume a sufficient amount of fruits and vegetables while staying within energy needs. Two cups of fruit and 2½ cups of vegetables per day are recommended for a reference 2,000-calorie intake, with higher or lower amounts depending on the calorie level. • Choose a variety of fruits and vegetables each day. In particular, select from all five vegetable subgroups (dark green, orange, legumes, starchy vegetables, and other vegetables) several times a week. • Consume 3 or more ounce-equivalents of whole-grain products per day, with the rest of the recommended grains coming from enriched or whole-grain products. In general, at least half the grains should come from whole grains. • Consume 3 cups per day of fat-free or low-fat milk or equivalent milk products.

continued

TABLE 1-1 Continued

Fats	• Consume less than 10 percent of calories from saturated fatty acids and less than 300 mg/day of cholesterol, and keep trans fatty acid consumption as low as possible. • Keep total fat intake between 20 to 35 percent of calories, with most fats coming from sources of polyunsaturated and monounsaturated fatty acids, such as fish, nuts, and vegetable oils. • When selecting and preparing meat, poultry, dry beans, and milk or milk products, make choices that are lean, low-fat, or fat-free. • Limit intake of fats and oils high in saturated and/or trans-fatty acids, and choose products low in such fats and oils.
Carbohydrates	• Choose fiber-rich fruits, vegetables, and whole grains often. • Choose and prepare foods and beverages with little added sugars or caloric sweeteners, such as amounts suggested by the USDA Food Guide and the DASH Eating Plan. • Reduce the incidence of dental caries by practicing good oral hygiene and consuming sugar- and starch-containing foods and beverages less frequently.
Sodium and potassium	• Consume less than 2,300 mg of sodium (approximately 1 teaspoon of salt) per day. • Choose and prepare foods with little salt. At the same time, consume potassium-rich foods, such as fruits and vegetables.
Alcoholic beverages	• Those who choose to drink alcoholic beverages should do so sensibly and in moderation—defined as the consumption of up to one drink per day for women and up to two drinks per day for men. • Alcoholic beverages should not be consumed by some individuals, including those who cannot restrict their alcohol intake, women of childbearing age who may become pregnant, pregnant and lactating women, children and adolescents, individuals taking medications that can interact with alcohol, and those with specific medical conditions. • Alcoholic beverages should be avoided by individuals engaging in activities that require attention, skill, or coordination, such as driving or operating machinery.
Food safety	• To avoid microbial foodborne illness: —Clean hands, food contact surfaces, and fruits and vegetables. Meat and poultry should not be washed or rinsed. —Separate raw, cooked, and ready-to-eat foods while shopping for, preparing, or storing foods. —Cook foods to a safe temperature to kill microorganisms. —Chill (refrigerate) perishable food promptly and defrost foods properly. —Avoid raw (unpasteurized) milk or any products made from unpasteurized milk, raw or partially cooked eggs or foods containing raw eggs, raw or undercooked meat and poultry, unpasteurized juices, and raw sprouts.

SOURCE: DHHS/USDA, 2005.

develop wellness policies to address the problem of childhood overweight and obesity (*Child Nutrition and WIC Reauthorization Act of 2004*. Public Law 108–265. 108th Congress. 2004). The wellness policy contains four basic components: nutrition education goals, physical activity goals, nutrition guidelines, and other school-based activities. The law specifies that the wellness policy include "nutrition guidelines selected by the local education agency for all foods available on each school campus under the local education agency during the school day with the objectives of promoting health and reducing childhood obesity." Although school districts across the country have taken steps toward meeting wellness policy requirements, these policies show great variability. Additionally, individual districts have expressed interest in being provided with information to enhance their understanding of nutrition and health issues and to assist them in developing strong wellness policies.

THE COMMITTEE'S TASK

In the FY 2005 Consolidated Appropriations, House Report 108–792, Congress directed the Centers for Disease Control and Prevention (CDC) to initiate a study with the Institute of Medicine (IOM) to review evidence and make recommendations about appropriate nutrition standards for the availability, sale, content, and consumption of foods at school, with attention to foods offered in competition with federally reimbursable meals and snacks. An ad hoc committee of the IOM was thus convened and charged to

- draw on literature regarding the availability, nutritional profile, and risks (including substitution) of school foods and beverages, including recent work by the Government Accountability Office, as appropriate;
- synthesize lessons learned from relevant research, development of federal nutrition standards for the National School Lunch and Breakfast Programs, and experience from the development of state- and local-based standards for foods and beverages offered outside federally reimbursable meals and snacks;
- consider whether a single set of nutrition standards is appropriate for elementary, middle, and high schools, or if more than one set is needed;
- develop nutrition standards based on nutritional science for foods and beverages, other than federally reimbursable meals and snacks, offered in school;
- consider how to ensure that foods and beverages offered in schools contribute to an overall healthful eating environment; and
- develop benchmarks to guide future evaluation studies of the application of the standards.

Approach to the Task

To address its charge, the committee reviewed available evidence from the current literature and from public workshop presentations by recognized experts (see Appendix E), developed guiding principles, and deliberated on issues relevant to its charge.

The committee reviewed literature, but did not conduct its own systematic, comprehensive evidence-based review. One challenge faced by the committee was interpreting limited evidence. Where evidence was inconclusive, the committee used its judgment to inform its interpretation of findings. An important starting point for the committee was the *Dietary Guidelines for Americans* (DHHS/USDA, 2005), together with the technical report of the Dietary Guidelines Advisory Committee (DHHS/USDA, 2004). The DGA is an evidence-based guideline that is a source of dietary health information for policymakers, nutrition educators, and health providers.

For areas not addressed in the DGA, such as caffeine and nonnutritive sweeteners, the committee conducted searches of original literature and reviews of these topics, including reports from the Government Accountability Office (GAO) on competitive foods in schools (GAO, 2005). The committee also recognized the importance of cost, but did not conduct an economic analysis of the recommended standards because it is beyond the scope of the report.

The committee was asked to provide benchmarks to evaluate programs. Because of the complexity of the issues, multiplicity of stakeholders, and lack of availability of data necessary to establish firm estimates and baselines, the committee lacked evidence and resources to address this task in detail with confidence. It did, however, put forward general guidelines for implementing the recommended standards and following up on the progress of implementation.

Organization of the Report

This report is organized into seven chapters. Chapter 1 describes the committee's task and introduces its guiding principles. Chapter 2 reviews nutrition-related health concerns that involve school-age children and adolescents. Chapter 3 describes the school environment and organizational structure and how these relate to federally reimbursable school meals and snacks, and competitive foods and beverages. Chapter 4 provides an in-depth discussion of foods and beverages offered outside the federally reimbursable school meals and the role of industry in the design and distribution of competitive foods in schools. Chapter 5 provides the committee's recommendations and Chapter 6 presents options for the implementation of the recommendations. The report references are listed in Chapter 7. Background and additional material are provided in the appendixes.

GUIDING PRINCIPLES

In response to the statement of task, the committee produced a set of "Guiding Principles" to effect development of nutritional standards for foods offered outside federally reimbursable meals and snacks. These principles are highlighted in Box 1-1 and described in detail below.

BOX 1-1
Guiding Principles

To initiate the study process, the committee developed a set of principles to guide their deliberations.

The committee recognizes that:

1. The present and future health and well-being of school-age children are profoundly affected by dietary intake and the maintenance of a healthy weight.

2. Schools contribute to current and lifelong health and dietary patterns and are uniquely positioned to model and reinforce healthful eating behaviors in partnership with parents, teachers, and the broader community.

3. Because foods and beverages available on the school campus represent significant caloric intake, they should be designed to meet nutrition standards.

4. Foods and beverages have health effects beyond those related to vitamins, minerals, and other known individual components.

5. Implementation of nutrition standards for foods and beverages offered in schools will likely require clear policies; technical and financial support; a monitoring, enforcement, and evaluation program; and new food and beverage products.

The committee intends that:

6. The federally reimbursable school nutrition programs will be the primary source of foods and beverages offered at school.

7. All foods and beverages offered on the school campus will contribute to an overall healthful eating environment.

8. Nutrition standards will be established for foods and beverages offered outside the federally reimbursable school nutrition programs.

9. The recommended nutrition standards will be based on the *Dietary Guidelines for Americans*, with consideration given to other relevant science-based resources.

10. The nutrition standards will apply to foods and beverages offered to all school-age children (generally ages 4 through 18 years) with consideration given to the developmental differences between children in elementary, middle, and high schools.

---

rationale for each Guiding Principle is presented below:

1. **The present and future health and well-being of school-age children are profoundly affected by dietary intake and the maintenance of a healthy weight.**

Although a healthy diet is important throughout life, research indicates that many children and adolescents have poor eating habits that fall far short of meeting recommended dietary guidelines. Poor eating habits also result in increased lifelong health risks such as overweight and obesity, diabetes, high cholesterol, high blood pressure, lowered immune resistance, iron deficiency anemia, some types of cancer, osteoporosis, and dental caries. However, childhood offers an enormous opportunity to provide a solid foundation for establishing healthful lifelong eating patterns. Taking advantage of this opportunity to improve the quality of children's diets is essential to the promotion of a healthier and more productive society.

2. **Schools contribute to current and lifelong health and dietary patterns and are uniquely positioned to model and reinforce healthful eating behaviors in partnership with parents, teachers, and the broader community.**

Fifty million 5- to 19-year-old children attend elementary and secondary schools, a number which represents more than 80 percent of all children in the United States (Gerald and Hussar, 2003; U.S. Census Bureau, 2006). Most children attend school for about 9 months per year from kindergarten through 12th grade. Where preschool is offered, some begin school at 3 to 4 years of age. Because children spend a large amount of time each day at school, they also consume a significant portion of their daily food intake at school. Although schools alone cannot address all the nutritional needs of children, they nonetheless play an important role in establishing short- and long-term dietary habits. Therefore, it is imperative for schools to promote good nutrition through healthful school meals and by ensuring that other foods and beverages available to students throughout the school campus contribute to a healthy diet.

Promoting children's health through public health initiatives, from ensuring that students are immunized to improving their nutritional status through the NSLP, is and will continue to be a fundamental aspect of the U.S. public school system. This basic tenet has been confirmed in numerous federal agency reports and consensus documents such as *Healthy People 2010* (DHHS, 2000), *Preventing Childhood Obesity: Health in the Balance* (IOM, 2005b), *Food Marketing to Children and Youth: Threat or Opportunity?* (IOM, 2006), and *School Health Services and Programs* (Lear et al., 2006). In addition, school food has been a concern of the federal government since the Depression era. Congress and the U.S. Department of Agriculture (USDA) set detailed standards for school lunch and breakfast programs, and the federal government invests about $10 billion a year in them.

In addition, the presence of children in a school setting for many hours each day provides a multitude of opportunities for modeling and reinforcing healthful eating behaviors. There are opportunities in formal classroom nutrition education programs as a component of other academic courses such as math, language arts, and science; and in classroom hands-on experiences with the preparation and consumption of food.

Opportunities to model and reinforce healthful eating behaviors are also available through the offering of healthful foods and beverages in the school meal and snack programs as part of à la carte sales in the cafeteria and throughout the school campus (e.g., in vending machines, school stores and clubs, and in the classroom). Although there are many influences on students' eating habits (both positive and negative) and numerous settings outside of school where children eat and drink, the school setting is the place in which the most curriculums are provided, and healthful behaviors and positive attitudes can be modeled and reinforced. This should apply to the healthfulness of foods and beverages as much as it does to the quality of curriculums, textbooks, science-based books, and rules of behavior.

3. **Because foods and beverages available on the school campus represent significant caloric intake, they should be designed to meet nutrition standards.**

Because children spend a large amount of time at school, they often consume a large proportion of their foods and beverages there—estimates range from 19 to 50 percent or more of total calories (Gleason and Suitor, 2001). School meal programs have been increasingly successful (Fox et al., 2001), and are on a continuing trajectory to be even more successful in promoting healthful foods and beverages. However, schools today offer students many opportunities to consume foods and beverages outside the school meal programs and throughout the school day. For example, students have access to various other food and beverages sold as à la carte in the cafeteria, and other competitive foods and beverages available via vending machines, school stores, classroom parties, and fundraisers.

The School Health Policies and Programs Study (SHPPS) found that 43 percent of elementary schools, 74 percent of middle schools, and 98 percent of high schools had vending machines, school snack bars, and other food and beverage sources outside of the school meal programs (Wechsler et al., 2001). A 2005 survey conducted by the U.S. Department of Education found that 94 percent of elementary schools offered foods and beverages for sale outside of school meal programs (Parsad and Lewis, 2006). The GAO found that nine out of ten schools offered competitive foods and beverages through à la carte cafeteria lines, vending machines, and school stores (GAO, 2005).

Although many schools and districts are improving competitive food and beverage offerings, they have a long way to go in promoting healthful choices. The SHPPS found that the most commonly consumed competitive foods and beverages were high in sugar, fat, and salt (Wechsler et al., 2001). Other studies also have found that à la carte offerings are of lesser nutritional quality (French et al., 2003; Harnack et al., 2000; Probart et al., 2005).

4. **Foods and beverages have health effects beyond those related to vitamins, minerals, and other known individual components.**

The 2005 DGA (DHHS/USDA, 2005) and MyPyramid (USDA, 2005) provide advice to help Americans choose a healthful diet. As stated, "The intent of the Dietary Guidelines is to summarize and synthesize knowledge regarding individual nutrients and food components into recommendations for a pattern of eating that can be adopted by the public" (DHHS/USDA, 2005). The DGA further states, "A basic premise of the Dietary Guidelines is that nutrient needs should be met primarily through consuming foods. Foods provide an array of nutrients and other compounds that may have beneficial effects on health" (DHHS/USDA, 2005). This is especially important to consider in the school setting where lifelong habits will be encouraged and developed.

A growing body of evidence suggests the important role that fruits, vegetables, whole grains, and nonfat and low-fat dairy play in our diet. The recommended standards comprise both nutrient- and food-based standards to remain consistent with the DGA and to recognize the importance of consuming nutrients through foods and beverages.

5. **Implementation of nutrition standards for foods and beverages offered in schools will likely require clear policies; technical and financial support; a monitoring, enforcement, and evaluation program; and new food and beverage products.**

Currently, there are many school, school district, and state policies on foods and beverages available outside the federally reimbursable school nutrition programs. Some standards are detailed and others are more general. Moreover, in some settings where competitive foods and beverages are offered, and at some grade levels, there are no policies at all. Thus, for nutrition standards to be implemented in schools that choose to allow these foods and beverages, policy changes at the school and school district level, and sometimes at the state and federal level, may be necessary.

In addition, school and school district staffs have varying levels of experience putting nutrition standards into practice. Some may require technical assistance and additional funding to implement these changes. They will also need the assistance of food and beverage suppliers to provide products that comply with the standards. Furthermore, to ensure that the standards are more than mere words on paper, responsibility must be assigned to personnel in the school or school district for monitoring the implementation and enforcement of the recommendations and for program evaluation. Finally, it will be important for school personnel, parents, and other parties to have access to information on implementation of the standards and patterns of food and beverage consumption in local settings.

6. **The federally reimbursable school nutrition programs will be the primary source of foods and beverages offered at school.**
Current nutrition standards for school meals are based on the 1995 Dietary Guidelines and are being revised and updated to meet the 2005 guidelines (USDA, 2006). The standards require that breakfast and lunch menus, when averaged over a school week, meet the following:

- Limit total fat intake to no more than 30 percent of calories and saturated fat to less than 10 percent of calories
- Provide one-third of the Recommended Dietary Allowance for protein, iron, calcium, and vitamins A and C for lunch and one-fourth for breakfast
- Steadily decrease the level of sodium
- Provide a varied menu, abundant in fruits, vegetables, and whole grains

School meals are evaluated according to these standards, and national studies show that schools are moving steadily toward compliance (Fox et al., 2001).

Children who participate in the school meal programs consume more fruits, vegetables, and dairy products compared to those who do not (Gleason and Suitor, 2001). In addition, students participating in the school meal program are likely to have a better sense of what constitutes a nutritionally complete meal. Given the nutritional benefits of consuming school meals, they should serve as the main source of nutrition in school. The committee recognizes that some school children may depend on home food sources for some or all meals and snacks consumed during the day.

7. **All foods and beverages offered on the school campus will contribute to an overall healthful eating environment.**
In addition to the prevalence of foods and beverages high in fat, sugar, and salt, evidence also suggests that the consumption of such products displaces the consumption of fruits, vegetables, and other healthful foods in children's diets (Cullen and Zakeri, 2004; Kubik et al., 2003; Templeton et al., 2005).

The current availability of foods and beverages sold outside the school meal programs (Wechsler et al., 2001) and their overall poor nutritional quality contribute to the increased consumption of less healthful foods and the overconsumption of calories (Cullen and Zakeri, 2004; Kubik et al., 2003; Templeton et al., 2005).

For schools to take full advantage of their unique position to model and reinforce healthy eating behaviors, the nutrition standards established consider foods and beverages offered in all venues and throughout the school day.

8. **Nutrition standards will be established for foods and beverages offered outside the federally reimbursable school nutrition programs.**

In addition to the school meals, which are planned to achieve nutrition standards over a school week, students have opportunities within the cafeteria and throughout the school campus to consume a variety of foods and beverages. These widely accessible items are often high in fat, sugar, and salt, making it increasingly difficult for children to eat a healthful overall diet.

Most children do not consume a diet consistent with the DGA and many have access, often unlimited and unsupervised, to a variety of items outside school meal programs. Therefore, it is essential to establish a set of nutrition standards for these competitive foods and beverages in order to increase a student's likelihood of meeting the DGA recommendations.

9. **The recommended nutrition standards will be based on the *Dietary Guidelines for Americans*, with consideration given to other relevant science-based resources.**

The DGA (DHHS/USDA, 2005) represents the most comprehensive U.S. evidence review of current scientific literature on diet and health, and it serves as the basis for federally funded school food and nutrition education programs. Other relevant resources considered included the IOM reports *Preventing Childhood Obesity: Health in the Balance* (IOM, 2005b), *Food Marketing to Children and Youth: Threat or Opportunity?* (IOM, 2006), *Progress in Preventing Childhood Obesity: How Do We Measure Up?* (IOM, 2007), the Dietary Reference Intake reports (IOM, 1997, 1998, 2000, 2001, 2002/2005, 2005a), and the report series on diet and health produced by the Food and Agriculture Organization of the United Nations/World Health Organization (WHO, 2003). In addition, position statements from professional nutrition and health associations, such as the American Academy of Pediatrics, also may be considered. Although contextual factors such as the ability of the marketplace and the school administration to respond to the recommendations may be weighed, the main objective is to improve the health of children.

10. **The nutrition standards will apply to foods and beverages offered to all school-age children (generally ages 4 through 18 years), with consideration given to the developmental differences between children in elementary, middle, and high schools.**

The DGA (DHHS/USDA, 2005) applies to all adults and children over the age of 2 years. However, there are key developmental differences between elementary and secondary school children. These differences include higher requirements for calcium and energy during adolescence, a gap between requirements and actual consumption for several nutrients and food groups among adolescents, and the limited ability of elementary school children to make appropriate choices among multiple food and beverage offerings.

Although the committee recognizes that there is individual variability among students even within a given educational level or grade, the standards are based on the DGA, which apply across the board to all Americans—regardless of weight status or activity level. Therefore, for students who are very active on most or all days of the week and who require more calories, the foods and beverages recommended are still appropriate.

SUMMARY

The quality of nutritional intake has a profound effect on a range of health issues. Improving childhood nutritional status improves the future health of the nation by diminishing individual risk factors for chronic diseases that include type 2 diabetes, cardiovascular disease, osteoporosis, and dental caries. These issues are examined in more detail in the following chapter.

2

Nutrition-Related Health Concerns, Dietary Intakes, and Eating Behaviors of Children and Adolescents

INTRODUCTION

Good nutrition during childhood and adolescence is essential for growth and development, health and well-being, and the prevention of some chronic diseases. Yet many American children's diets fall considerably short of recommended dietary standards. Furthermore, poor diet and physical inactivity, resulting in an energy imbalance, are the most important factors contributing to the increase in obesity in childhood. Obesity is the most pressing challenge to nutritional health in this first decade of the 21st century (CDC, 1999). The major nutrition issues among children and adolescents have shifted from nutrient deficiency diseases, common in the first half of the 20th century, to concerns today about overconsumption, poor dietary quality, and food choices. However, food insecurity remains a concern among the poor (Briefel and Johnson, 2004). This chapter provides an overview on nutrition-related health concerns, current dietary and nutrient intakes, and dietary trends over the past 20–40 years for children and adolescents.

Importance of Healthful Dietary Behaviors in School-Age Children and Adolescents

During childhood and adolescence, good nutrition and dietary behaviors are important to achieve full growth potential and appropriate body composition, to promote health and well-being, and to reduce the risk of chronic diseases in adulthood. Children require sufficient energy, protein, and other nutrients for growth as well as maintenance of body functions. Nutrient needs tend to parallel rates of growth. Growth continues at a steady rate during childhood, then accelerates during adolescence, creating increases in nutrient needs to support the rapid growth rate and increase in lean body mass and body size (Story et al., 2002a). During puberty, adolescents achieve the final 15 to 20 percent of stature, gain 50 percent of adult body weight, and accumulate up to 40 percent of skeletal mass (Story et al., 2002a). Inadequate intakes of energy, protein, or certain micronutrients will be reflected in slow growth rates, delayed sexual maturation, inadequate bone mass, and low body reserves of micronutrients (Story et al., 2002a).

In addition to the impact on growth and development, children's diets are important to ensure overall health and well-being. Dietary practices of children and adolescents affect their risk for a number of health problems, including obesity, iron deficiency, and dental caries. Inadequate nutrition also lowers resistance to infectious disease, and may adversely affect the ability to function at peak mental and physical ability. Obesity in children and adolescents is associated with a number of immediate health risks, such as high blood pressure, type 2 diabetes (T2D), metabolic syndrome, sleep disturbances, orthopedic problems, and psychosocial problems (Daniels, 2006; IOM, 2005b). Furthermore, obese adolescents are likely to remain overweight as adults (IOM, 2005b). Indeed, longitudinal epidemiological studies provide evidence that obesity, hypercholesterolemia, and hypertension track from childhood into adulthood and lifestyle choices such as diet and excess caloric intake influence these conditions (Gidding et al., 2005).

There is concern about long-term health as certain dietary patterns, developed in childhood and carried into adulthood, result in an increased risk for chronic diseases, such as obesity, heart disease, osteoporosis, and some types of cancer later in life. Some of the physiological processes that lead to diet-related chronic diseases have their onset during childhood. For example, studies indicate that the process of atherosclerosis begins in childhood (Gidding et al., 2005). Nutritional factors contribute significantly to the burden of preventable illnesses and premature deaths in the United States (DHHS, 2000). Four of the ten leading causes of death in adults are diet related: diabetes, coronary heart disease (CHD), certain cancers, and strokes. Diet is also associated with osteoporosis. Dietary factors also contribute to reproductive health, e.g., adequate consumption of folic acid to prevent neural tube defects in infants.

Dietary patterns are influenced by behavioral choices and environmental factors. It may be easier to change children's health behavior than adults' behavior. Childhood offers the opportunity to provide the solid foundation needed for healthful lifelong eating patterns. The importance of applying a life-course approach, starting early in life, to the prevention of chronic diseases and obesity has also been emphasized (WHO, 2003). A principal goal of public health is to give people the best chance to enjoy a long and healthy life. Children represent the nation's present and its future.

OVERVIEW OF CHILDREN'S NUTRITION-RELATED HEALTH CONCERNS

The rising rate of obesity in children has become a major health concern, both because of its impact on childhood health and its potential effect on the development of chronic disease in adulthood. Obesity status is usually indicated by the body mass index (BMI), which is a measure in which weight is adjusted for height. More specifically, BMI is defined as weight in kilograms divided by height in meters squared. For adults, weight status is based on the absolute BMI level, and in children BMI percentile. BMI measurements in children adjust the children's weight and stature by their age and gender. In this report, the term "obesity" is used to refer to children and adolescents who have a BMI at or above the age and sex-specific 95th percentile of the BMI charts developed by the Centers for Disease Control and Prevention (CDC) in 2000. Those children and adolescents who have a BMI between the 85th and 95th percentile for age and sex are termed at risk for obesity. In most children and youth, a BMI level at or above the 95th percentile indicates elevated body fat and reflects the presence or risk of related chronic disease (IOM, 2005b, 2007).

Trends in Childhood Obesity

Childhood obesity has been increasing steadily, particularly during the past two decades. The number of children above the 95th percentile of weight for height has tripled among those in the age bracket of 12 to 19 years, rising from 5 percent in 1976–80 to 17 at present (Ogden et al., 2002, 2006). The National Health and Nutrition Examination Survey (NHANES) III (1988–1994) found an increase from 7 to 11 percent in obesity for 6- to 11-year-old children, compared to NHANES II a decade earlier (1976–1980) (Ogden et al., 2002). Further NHANES survey data (1999–2004) confirmed the continued rise in obesity. Another 15 percent of children and adolescents are estimated to be at risk for obesity (85th to 95th percentile), making a third of children and adolescents obese or at-risk for obesity (Ogden et al., 2002, 2006). These trends are shown in Figure 2-1.

Although childhood obesity has increased in every demographic population group in the United States, some have been more affected than oth-

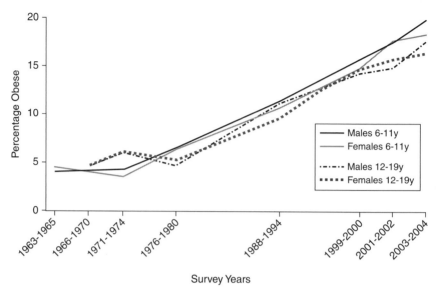

Survey Years

FIGURE 2-1 Trends in child and adolescent obesity in males and females aged 6–19 years.

NOTE: Obesity is defined as a body mass index (BMI) at or above the age- and gender-specific 95th-percentile cutoff points from the 2004 Centers for Disease Control and Prevention BMI Charts. The data on which this figure is based may have a standard error of 20 to 30 percent.

SOURCE: Derived from IOM, 2005b; Ogden et al., 2002/2006.

ers. For example, using data from the 2003–2004 NHANES, Ogden et al. (2006) reported obesity rates of 19 and 16 percent for white boys and girls respectively, aged 6–19 years. The rates of obesity in African American children were 18 percent for boys and 26 percent for girls, and among Mexican-American children, the rates were 22 percent for boys and 17 percent for girls. Other research has shown similar or higher rates of obesity (Sorof et al., 2004). In samples of minority children from three states, 29 percent were obese and another 19.8 percent were at risk for obesity (Jago et al., 2006). In New York City nearly half of 2,700 students surveyed were at risk for obesity (Thorpe et al., 2004). The average rate of obesity in this student population was 31 percent among Hispanic (36 percent among boys), 23 percent among African American, 16 percent among white, and 14 percent among Asian children (Thorpe et al., 2004). Childhood obesity status tracks into adulthood obesity status (Deshmukh-Taskar et al., 2006; Raitakari et al., 2005).

Associations Between Obesity and Chronic Disease

The increased prevalence of obesity in childhood is of concern because of the strong association between obesity and cardiovascular disease risk, hypertension, dyslipidemia, and T2D that begins in childhood and continues into adulthood.

Cardiovascular Disease

Cardiovascular disease (CVD) is the leading cause of death and disability in the U.S., responsible for some 500,000 deaths a year. Most CVD is the result of the process of atherosclerosis whereby plaque builds up in blood vessels. About 50 percent of CVD is related to coronary artery disease. Although the clinical effects of the process do not usually show up until middle age, atherosclerosis begins in childhood and the extent of atherosclerotic change in childhood and young adulthood is correlated with elevated risk in adults (Rodriguez et al., 2006; Williams et al., 2002).

Risk factors for CVD, such as elevated serum cholesterol and blood pressure occur with increased frequency in obese children and adolescents compared to children with a normal weight. In a population-based sample, approximately 60 percent of obese children aged 5 to 10 years had at least one physiological CVD risk factor, such as elevated total cholesterol, triglycerides, insulin, or blood pressure, and 25 percent had two or more CVD risk factors (Freedman et al., 1999). These risk factors are related in some degree to lifestyle factors such as diet and physical activity. The American Heart Association concludes that existing evidence indicates that primary prevention of atherosclerotic disease should begin in childhood (Williams et al., 2002).

Hypertension

Hypertension contributes substantially to CVD, renal failure, and premature death. The diagnosis of hypertension in children and adolescents is based on the distribution of blood pressure measurement in healthy children. Those with an average systolic or diastolic blood pressure above the 95th percentile for age, gender, and height on three separate occasions are considered to be hypertensive, while those between the 90th and 95th percentile are considered high normal or prehypertensive and are at increased risk for hypertension (AAP, 2004a). NHANES 1999–2000 found that 8 percent of children and adolescents aged 12 to 19 years had hypertension. Recent studies with participants who were predominantly minority and, on average, higher in weight, have shown around 20 to 25 percent of children with hypertension or prehypertension. The rates increase with higher BMIs, from 14 percent of those with normal BMI percentile, to 27 percent of those at risk for obesity, to 39 percent of those who are obese (Jago et al., 2006). This finding differs by ethnic group, ranging from 25 percent among Hispanic to 16 percent among Asian children (Sorof et al., 2004). The relative risk for hypertension continues to be significant for obesity even when ethnicity, gender, and other factors are controlled. Comparing rates between the 1988–1994 and 1999–2000 NHANES shows that hypertension among children and adolescents has increased over time. This increase is partially accounted for by the increase in obesity (Muntner et al., 2004).

Diabetes

Type 2 diabetes is a complex glucose and insulin metabolic disease that can lead to serious consequences such as diabetic retinopathy, peripheral neuropathy, and kidney failure. Diabetes also increases the risk of atherosclerosis with its attendant risks of stroke, heart attack, and hypertension. Obesity in children is a major element in insulin resistance and is thus a risk factor for T2D. Type 2 diabetes has been considered an adult disease, commonly diagnosed in persons 40–74 years of age. However, the diagnosis of T2D has increased dramatically in children and adolescents and is related to body fatness.

Although the rate in years past was about 5 to 10 percent of the population diagnosed with the disease, it is now estimated that, for individuals born in the U.S. after 2000, the lifetime risk of being diagnosed with T2D is 30 percent for boys and 40 percent for girls if obesity rates level off (Narayan et al., 2003). The lifetime risk of developing diabetes is even higher in some ethnic minorities at birth and at all ages. Indeed, in some communities, diabetes will become normative, that is, more individuals will have it than not. These high rates of diagnosis in children and adolescents will have considerable public health consequences: the longer a person has the disease, the greater the risk of complications. This will have an impact on schools, colleges, and workplaces, as each setting will have to deal with the increasing effects of this severe and debilitating disease in the form of days lost from school or work, discomfort, ill health, disabilities, and increased medical visits. In addition, the cost of treating diabetes, which has been estimated at $132 billion a year, will increase as today's children and adolescents reach adulthood (American Diabetes Association, 2003).

Metabolic Syndrome

Metabolic syndrome is a constellation of clinical findings, including abdominal obesity, high blood pressure, dyslipidemia, and high glucose levels, that confers increased risk for CVD and T2D. Metabolic syndrome is also called "syndrome X" and insulin resistance syndrome. An analysis of data from NHANES III (1988–1994) found that the overall prevalence of metabolic syndrome among all adolescents aged 12 to 19 years was 4.2 percent (6 percent in males and 2 percent in females). The syndrome was present in more than a fourth (28.7 percent) of obese adolescents, compared to 6.8 percent in adolescents at risk for obesity and 0.1 percent of those with a BMI below the 85th percentile (p <.001). Based on population-weighted estimates, this means that in the U.S. approximately 900,000 adolescents have metabolic syndrome (Cook et al., 2003). Another study found that the prevalence of metabolic syndrome increased with the severity of obesity and reached 50 percent in severely obese children and adolescents (Weiss et al., 2004). Other studies have shown clustering of components of metabolic syndrome with coronary and aortic atherosclerosis in young adults (Berenson et al., 1998).

Increasing childhood obesity rates affect not only individuals and their families, but also impose direct and indirect economic costs in the forms of lost productivity, disability, morbidity, and premature death. States and communities will have to allocate new resources to prevent and treat the various metabolic syndrome comorbidities. Indeed, the great advances in the nation's health as a result of the decline in nutritional deficiencies and the promise of advances in biomedical discoveries may be offset by the burden of illness, disability, and death resulting from metabolic syndrome and comorbidities. Therefore, schools have the opportunity and responsibility to address this nutritional and social problem within the school-age population.

Bone Health and Osteoporosis

Osteoporosis is a complex disorder with many contributing factors. Osteoporosis is characterized by low bone mass and microarchitectural deterioration of bone tissue, resulting in fragility and an increased risk of fracture (WHO, 2003). Osteoporotic fractures are a major cause of morbidity and disability in older people. An estimated 10 million Americans over age 50 have osteoporosis and another 34 million are at risk (DHHS, 2004a). Each year an estimated 1.5 million Americans suffer an osteoporotic-related fracture. One out of every two women over 50 years of age will have an osteoporosis-related fracture in her lifetime, with risk of fracture increasing with age (DHHS, 2004a). Health-care costs associated with osteoporotic fractures are estimated at $12–18 billion per year in 2002 dollars (DHHS, 2004a). Because of the expected increase in the number of individuals in the age range of highest risk, the incidence of hip fractures in the United States may triple by the year 2040. Although bone disease often strikes later in life, the importance of maintaining bone health and early prevention is now well recognized. It is believed that with good nutrition (especially adequate intake of calcium and vitamin D) and physical activity throughout life, individuals can achieve and maintain good bone health and significantly reduce the risk of bone disease and fractures (DHHS, 2004a).

Because of the importance of bone health in childhood, osteoporosis can be viewed as a pediatric disorder that manifests itself later in life. Late childhood and the adolescent years provide the window of opportunity to influence lifelong bone health. Approximately 45 percent of the adult skeleton is acquired between the ages of 9 and 17 years (Weaver and Heaney, 2006). Approximately 60 to 80 percent of bone mass is genetically determined, but hormones and lifestyle factors play a role in determining peak bone mass, which is typically achieved by the time an individual reaches the mid-teens to early 20s (DHHS, 2004a). Development of a higher peak bone mass during the adolescent years likely protects against age-related bone loss (DHHS, 2004a; Heaney et al., 2000; Weaver et al., 1999). Because the amount of bone accumulated during pubertal growth depends to some extent on the amount of calcium and vitamin D in the diet, low calcium intakes during skeletal formation may result in decreased bone mass (Heaney et al., 2000). Variations in calcium nutrition in late childhood and adolescence may account for a 5- to 10-percent difference in peak bone mass resulting in a difference of 25- to 50-percent of hip fracture incidence later in life (Heaney et al., 2000). Epidemiological evidence supports the hypothesis that low bone mass may be a contributing factor to fractures in children (Greer and Krebs, 2006).

Many studies have examined the association between calcium intake during childhood and adolescence and bone health. Of 52 calcium intervention studies, all but two showed a correlation between improved bone density at higher intakes, greater bone gain during growth, reduced bone loss in the elderly, or reduced fracture risk (Heaney, 2000). Maintaining adequate calcium intake during childhood and adolescence is critical to achieving peak bone mass (Greer and Krebs, 2006). As is discussed below, the majority of older children and adolescents do not reach the recommended intakes of calcium.

Iron Deficiency

Iron deficiency is the most common nutritional deficiency in the world. Iron deficiency represents a spectrum ranging from iron depletion, which causes no physiological impairments, to iron-deficiency anemia, which affects the functioning of several organ systems (CDC, 1998). Iron deficiency and anemia are known to impair psychomotor development, affect physical activity and work capacity, lower resistance to infection, and, in pregnant women, increase the risk of preterm delivery and delivering a low birth-weight infant (IOM, 2001). Iron deficiency has also been linked to poorer cognition and behavioral and learning problems among school-age children and adolescents (Grantham-McGregor and Ani, 2001; Halterman et al., 2001; Pollitt and Mathews, 1998). For example, one recent study investigated the relationship between iron deficiency and test scores among a nationally representative sample of school-age children and adolescents and found lower standardized math scores among iron-deficient children and adolescents, including those with iron deficiency without anemia (Halterman et al., 2001).

Iron deficiency is highest among toddlers, women of childbearing age, and pregnant women. Adolescents undergoing rapid growth periods are also at risk as iron requirements increase dramatically as a result of the expansion of total blood volume, the increase in lean body mass, and the onset of menses in young females (Beard, 2000). According to NHANES (1999–2000) data of all age groups, the prevalence of iron deficiency was highest (16 percent) among females aged 16–19 years. Among children and adolescents aged 12–15 years, 9 percent of females and 5 percent of males had iron deficiency (CDC, 2002). National data indicate that only one-fourth of all females of childbearing age meet the dietary recommendations for iron (15 mg/day). Primary prevention of iron deficiency means ensuring an adequate intake of iron (CDC, 1998). This includes selecting iron-rich foods and increasing consumption of foods that enhance iron absorption.

Dental Caries

Although dental caries (tooth decay) is largely preventable, it is the single most common chronic disease among American children and is twice as common among low-income compared to higher-income families (DHHS, 2004b). Low-income children have about 12 times more restricted activity days due to dental-related diseases than children from higher-income families. Pain due to untreated tooth decay can lead to problems in eating, speaking, and attending to learning (CDC/DHHS, 2006). The most recent NHANES data (1999–2002) found that, among all children aged 2 to 11 years, 41 percent had dental caries in primary teeth. There are disparities evident with children in lower-income households and African American, Hispanic, and American Indian children having a higher prevalence of dental problems (DHHS, 2000, 2004b). Among children and adolescents aged 6 to 19 years, 42 percent had dental caries in permanent teeth (Beltran-Aguilar et al., 2005). Topical fluoride in toothpaste, fluoridated water, and preventive dental care were found to have a significant impact on reduction of caries risk (Touger-Decker and van Loveren, 2003).

The role of diet in the etiology of dental caries is well established. There is consistently strong evidence that frequent consumption of sugar and other fermentable carbohydrates is associated with the development of caries (Lingstrom et al., 2003). Several reviews of the literature concluded a causal relationship between sugars and dental caries, although the relationship is not as strong as in the pre-fluoride era (Lingstrom et al., 2003;

Touger-Decker and van Loveren, 2003; WHO, 2003; Zero, 2004). Dietary habits of children remain a major component of the caries process (Dye et al., 2004). Furthermore, given the American propensity for frequent snacking, it is likely that many starch-containing processed foods also contribute to caries formation (Zero, 2004).

Other important factors in caries development are food form (e.g., liquid, solid, sticky), duration of exposure, nutrient composition, sequence of eating, potential to stimulate saliva, and presence of buffers (e.g., cheese, gum containing xylitol) (Moynihan and Petersen, 2004; Touger-Decker and Mobley, 2003). Risk factors related to food consumption include nocturnal meal consumption and frequent sugar consumption (Bankel et al., 2006), and the form of sugar-containing food (Marshall et al., 2007). Intake frequency of sugars is considered the most important dietary factor in caries development (Lingstrom et al., 2003; Moynihan and Petersen, 2004). Tooth erosion refers to the gradual loss of the outside, hard surface of the tooth due to chemical, not bacterial, processes (Touger-Decker and Mobley, 2003). Tooth erosion involving frequent intake of acidic foods and beverages weakens tooth integrity and further increases caries risk (Touger-Decker and Mobley, 2003). Tooth erosion is increasing in industrialized countries and is thought to be related to increased consumption of acidic beverages (e.g., soft drinks, sports drinks, and fruit juices) (Moynihan and Petersen, 2004). Because of the synergistic relationship between nutrition and oral health, and because nutrition is a critical component of oral health, the dietary habits of children and adolescents are needed to improve oral health.

Disordered Eating Behavior

Relative to many other public health problems, full-syndrome eating disorders are fairly rare among children and adolescents; however, they are a serious cause of morbidity and mortality in this group. More than 10 percent of individuals with anorexia nervosa admitted to university hospitals eventually die from the disorder (APA, 2000). Anorexia nervosa (characterized by self-starvation, weight loss, intense fear of weight gain, and body image distortion) (APA, 2000) affects less than 1 percent of adolescent females (Emans, 2000). Bulimia nervosa affects 1 to 5 percent of adolescent girls (Emans, 2000) and is characterized by binge eating and purging (APA, 2000). The onset of eating disorders often occurs during adolescence or early adulthood (Emans, 2000). About 5 to 10 percent of all adolescents with an eating disorder are male (APA, 2000).

Eating disorders are viewed as multifactor disorders with environmental and social factors, psychological predisposition, and biological and genetic predisposition. "Dieting" is a common entry point in both anorexia nervosa and bulimia nervosa, with the greatest risk being the group of severe dieters (Rome et al., 2003). Sociocultural and environmental factors as they relate to ideal body shape are thought to play an important role in the development of eating disorders. Eating disorders are more common in countries and cultures where female thinness is associated with attractiveness (Rome et al., 2003).

More common in the preadolescent and adolescent population are dieting and disordered eating behaviors. Dieting is a common and widespread practice especially among girls. Nationwide in 2005, 62 percent of high school girls (whites, 64 percent; African Americans, 53 percent; Hispanics, 64 percent) reported trying to lose weight during the 30 days preceding the survey. Thirty percent of high school boys were trying to lose weight (Eaton et al., 2006). Nearly 17 percent of females had gone without eating for 24 hours or more, 8 percent had taken diet pills, and 6 percent had induced vomiting or taken laxatives to lose weight during the previous 30 days (Eaton et al., 2006). Studies have shown that adolescent girls using unhealthy weight control behaviors consume fewer fruits, vegetables, and grains, and have lower intakes of calcium, iron, and other micronutrients compared to girls using healthy weight control methods or not dieting (Neumark-Sztainer et al., 2004; Story et al., 1998). A recent longitudinal study of adolescents found that dieting and unhealthy weight control behaviors among adolescents predicted weight gain, obesity status, disordered eating, and risk of eating disorder five years later (Neumark-Sztainer et al., 2006). These studies suggest that a shift is needed away from dieting and drastic weight control measures and toward lifelong healthful eating and weight control behaviors and physical activity behaviors.

DIETARY INTAKE AND CONSUMPTION PATTERNS OF CHILDREN AND ADOLESCENTS

Are Children's Diets Meeting the *Dietary Guidelines for Americans*?

The general dietary recommendations for those aged two years and older in the *Dietary Guidelines for Americans* (DGA) (DHHS/USDA, 2005) emphasize a diet that relies primarily on fruits and vegetables, whole grains, low-fat and nonfat dairy products, beans, fish, and lean meat. The guidelines stress meeting recommended dietary intakes within energy needs; consuming a variety of nutrient-dense foods and beverages; and limiting intakes of total, saturated, and trans fat, cholesterol, salt, and added sugars. The guidelines, as they pertain to children and adolescents, are consistent with other dietary recommendations for children and adolescents put forth by the American Heart Association (Gidding et al., 2005) and the American Academy of Pediatrics (AAP, 2004b).

Despite the importance of healthful eating patterns during childhood and adolescence, studies have consistently shown that this group has poor eating habits and does not meet dietary recommendations (Enns et al., 2002, 2003; Gleason and Suitor, 2001b; IOM, 2007; Moshfegh et al., 2005; Munoz et al., 1997). National data found that no more than 2 percent of children and adolescents met the Food Guide Pyramid recommendations, and 16 percent did not meet any of the food group recommendations (Munoz et al., 1997, 1998). Areas of concern include low intakes of fruits, vegetables, whole grains, fiber, and calcium-rich foods, and higher than recommended intakes of foods and beverages high in fat, sodium, and added sugars. The consumption of added sugars, saturated fats, and trans fats provides calories but few essential nutrients (DHHS/USDA, 2005). Current dietary patterns among children and adolescents lead to median intakes be-

---

BOX 2-1
Why Not Just Fortify? The Scientific Basis for
Promoting Fruits, Vegetables, and Whole Grains

The scientific basis for the Dietary Guidelines for Americans on fruits, vegetables, and whole grains is the epidemiological evidence that individuals who consume generous amounts of these foods on a regular basis have lower rates of cardiovascular disease (CVD), several cancers, diabetes, and other chronic diseases. These foods contain nutrients and phytochemicals that may lower chronic disease risk directly, or via established risk factors such as blood pressure and plasma cholesterol levels. In addition, diets high in these foods tend to have lower levels of fat, saturated fat, and cholesterol.

Clinical trials conducted with beta-carotene, vitamins A, C, and E, folic acid, and selenium (alone or in combination) examined the role of specific food components hypothesized to reduce chronic disease to determine if adding these components to other foods or supplements would have the same health benefits as consuming plant foods. However, the U.S. Preventive Services Task Force (USPSTF) concluded that the evidence is insufficient to recommend for or against the use of these food components as supplements for the prevention of chronic disease (USPSTF, 2003), and the National Institutes of Health Consensus Conference also concurs (NIH, 2006).

Underscoring the important scientific uncertainties concerning health effects of individual nutrients, it is noteworthy that the USPSTF recommends that beta-carotene not be used as a supplement, either alone or in combination, because of the evidence that it may increase the risk of lung cancer in high-risk individuals (USPSTF, 2003). More recent reports have confirmed the finding that these supplements are not effective in reducing cancer or CVD (Bjelakovic et al., 2004; Manson, 2003; Pham and Plakogiannis, 2005) and further suggested that high-dosage supplements of vitamin E may increase all-cause mortality (Miller

low recommended values for many nutrients (DHHS, 2000; DHHS/USDA, 2004; Gidding et al., 2005).

Emerging evidence for the health benefits of fruits, vegetables, and whole grains has important implications for strategies to improve children's diets. Specifically, it reinforces the importance of improving the overall quality of food intake rather than nutrient-specific strategies such as fortification and supplementation, and thus is consistent with the *Dietary Guidelines for Americans* (see Box 2-1). In addition, regular consumption of fortified beverages can contribute to the displacement of nutrient-dense beverages such as milk (see discussion of sweetened beverages below).

et al., 2005). Neuhouser et al. (2003) reported that the use of a high-dose beta-carotene and retinyl palmitate supplement negated the beneficial effects of a diet high in fruits and vegetables. The reasons for these unexpected findings remain unclear.

The conclusion drawn from negative findings in clinical trials is that the mechanisms by which plant foods decrease disease risk are likely the cumulative effect of numerous phytochemicals on multiple biochemical pathways, rather than the result of single nutrients or phytochemicals. An estimated 5,000+ phytochemicals have been identified in fruits, vegetables, and whole grains, but a large percentage still remain unknown and the study of their individual and combined effects of these on health and disease is just beginning (Jeffery, 2005; Liu, 2004). The concentration of individual and major classes of phytochemicals varies widely across different forms of fruits and vegetables and their biological activity does not necessarily correlate with the levels of nutrients in foods. For example, a 100-gram serving of apple (with peel) contains only 5.7 mg vitamin C, representing about 13 percent of the U.S. Recommended Dietary Allowance for 9- to 13-year olds. Yet the phytochemicals have antioxidant activity 250 times greater than that of the vitamin C alone (Liu, 2004). This suggests that, given current scientific knowledge, the use of nutrient content alone as a guide for the relative healthfulness of various foods or products is incomplete and potentially misleading.

In summary, the evolving understanding of plant foods highlights three key points. First, plant foods are compositionally complex. Second, the health benefits of plant foods appear to be closely related to their compositional complexity, not to individual components. Third, the levels of vitamins and minerals in foods do not necessarily correlate well with the other classes of beneficial components. These points reinforce the need for nutrition standards to go beyond the criteria of upper limits (for fat, saturated fat, etc.) and qualifying levels (for vitamins and minerals), and to place at least equal emphasis on the health benefits of fruits, vegetables, and whole grains.

Overview of Nutrient and Energy Intakes of Children and Adolescents

Nutrient Intakes

The Dietary Guidelines Advisory Committee (DGAC) reviewed the scientific literature and concluded that, based on dietary intake data or evidence of public health problems, intake levels of the following nutrients are of concern for children and adolescents: calcium, potassium, fiber, magnesium, vitamin E, and, for adolescent girls, iron and folate. The committee also found that in general, Americans consume too many calories and too much saturated and trans fat, cholesterol, added sugars, and salt (DHHS/USDA, 2004).

The most recent nationwide dietary intake data are for the years 2001–2002 and were collected as part of NHANES as 2 days of dietary data based on 24-hour recalls. NHANES is a multistage, stratified sample and was representative of the U.S. population. A recent report examined usual nutrient intakes from food compared to Dietary Reference Intakes[1] (DRIs) (Moshfegh et al., 2005) and found the following:

- Nearly all children 4–8 years old, and males 9–18 years old had adequate intakes (based on Estimated Average Requirement) of protein, folate, vitamin B6, thiamin, riboflavin, niacin, iron, zinc, copper, and phosphorus.
- The majority (>80 percent) of children and adolescents had inadequate dietary intakes of vitamin E. Vitamin A intakes were inadequate for one third of females aged 9–13 years and more than half of adolescents aged 14–18 years. Vitamin C intake was inadequate for one-fourth of males and 42 percent of females aged 14–18 years. Magnesium intake was inadequate among 9- to 13-year-olds.
- For dietary fiber and potassium, less than 3 percent of children and adolescents had intakes above the Adequate Intake level.
- Calcium intake was low for many children and adolescents. The following percentage of children had intakes below the Adequate Intake: 31 percent of children aged 4- to 8-years, 70 percent of males aged 9- to 18-years, and 92 percent of females aged 9- to 18-years.
- Females aged 14–18 years were at especially high risk of inadequate vitamin and mineral intakes, much higher than any of the other age and gender groups. For example, 54 percent had inadequate intake of vitamin A, 42 percent had inadequate intake of vitamin C, 91 percent had inadequate intake of magnesium, and 19 percent had inadequate intake of folate.

---

[1]The DRIs are a set of reference values for four nutrients established by the Food and Nutrition Board of the Institute of Medicine for use in assessing intakes of population groups (IOM, 1997, 1998, 2000, 2001, 2002/2005, 2005a).

The results of the NHANES 2001–2002 dietary survey are consistent with previous findings from the Continuing Survey of Food Intakes by Individuals (CSFII) national surveys (Gleason and Suitor, 2001b). In the 1994–1996 CSFII, most school-age children met the reference standards for the B vitamins (except folate), but many were at risk for inadequate intake of folate, magnesium, and vitamins A and E. Older children had lower intakes than younger ones and females had lower intakes than males. Large numbers of adolescent females failed to consume adequate amounts of vitamins and minerals. For most nutrients, racial/ethnic differences in intakes were small (Gleason and Suitor, 2001b). The results of these national studies point to concerns about the adequacy of the diets of today's children and adolescents.

Energy Intake

Energy is required to sustain body functions such as respiration, circulation, physical work, and core body temperature, and to meet growth requirements (IOM, 2002/2005). Energy intake should be commensurate with energy expenditure so as to achieve energy balance. Imbalances between intake and expenditure result in weight gain or loss. Energy expenditure depends on age and varies primarily as a function of body size and physical activity, both of which differ greatly among individuals. In children and adolescents, energy requirements include energy costs associated with growth needs and the deposition of tissue. However, the energy cost of growth is relatively low; for the adolescent pubertal growth spurt, it is only about 4 percent of the total energy requirement (IOM, 2002/2005).

Results of surveys of children's energy intakes present results that vary by gender and age. In NHANES III (1988–1994), the mean energy intakes for children 6–11 years of age were 2,146 kcal/day for boys and 1,793 kcal/day for girls. For adolescents 12–19 years of age, the mean energy intakes were 2,843 kcal/day for boys and 1,977 kcal/day for girls (Troiano et al., 2000). In NHANES, mean energy intakes changed little from the 1970s to 1988–1994, except for an increase in adolescent girls of 192 calories (Troiano et al., 2000). In the CSFII data for the same period, substantial increases were reported in the mean energy intakes of children and adolescents from the mid-1970s to the mid-1990s. Average energy intakes increased by 243 calories for adolescent boys and 113 calories for adolescent girls (Enns et al., 2003). For children aged 6–11 years, there were only modest increases of 100 calories for boys and about 30 calories for girls (Enns et al., 2002). However, as discussed below, a number of methodological studies provided evidence of underreporting in food intake surveys.

Excess weight gain or obesity may develop over several months from a relatively small daily excess (e.g., 50 to 100 calories/day) of calories consumed compared to calories expended (IOM, 2005b). Both excessive caloric intake and physical inactivity are likely contributors to the caloric imbalance that leads to excessive fat stores and obesity. A recent study modeled the magnitude of energy imbalance responsible for the increase in body weight among U.S. children during the periods 1988–1991 and 1999–2002. They found that a reduction in excess energy intake of 110–165 kcal/day could have prevented this increase (Wang et al., 2006).

Sodium Intake

Sodium is an essential mineral needed for normal fluid and electrolyte balance. Sodium homeostasis is maintained mostly through dietary intake and urinary excretion. The minimal metabolic requirement for sodium is estimated to be no more than 0.18 g/day (IOM, 2005a), although extremely low-sodium diets may lead to decreased intake of other essential minerals such as potassium, calcium, and magnesium. Sodium levels in blood and tissues can be conserved in conditions of low intake through reduced excretion in urine and sweat (Allan and Wilson, 1971; Allsopp et al., 1998).

Increased sodium intake is associated with elevated blood pressure, which in turn is a risk factor for cardiovascular and renal diseases. A dose-dependent but nonlinear relationship has been shown between sodium intake and blood pressure (Alderman, 2002). Genetic factors may increase sodium sensitivity and contribute to cardiovascular risk associated with high sodium intake (Franco and Oparil, 2006).

The bulk of the evidence supporting associations between sodium intake and blood pressure has been derived from studies on adults. Similar associations between sodium intake and increased blood pressure in children are not as well documented, although there is strong evidence to support an association between low sodium intake early in life and lower blood pressure in childhood and into adulthood (Geleijnse et al., 1990, 1997; Martin et al., 2003) and observational evidence to support that blood pressure levels track from childhood into adulthood (Bao et al., 1995; Dekkers et al., 2002; Gillman et al., 1993; Van Lenthe et al., 1994). Evidence from observational studies, randomized clinical trials, and longitudinal studies, however, is inconclusive about an association between reduction of dietary sodium and decreased blood pressure in children and adolescents (IOM, 2005a). Taken together, this evidence suggests that elevated blood pressure during childhood increases the risk for subsequent cardiovascular disease.

Dietary sodium is derived primarily from salt (sodium chloride) and food processing ingredients (e.g., sodium bicarbonate, monosodium glutamate, sodium phosphate, and sodium benzoate). The DGA (DHHS/USDA, 2005) recommendations for those age 2 years and above include

- consuming less than 2,300 mg (approximately 1 teaspoon of salt) per day; and

• choosing and preparing foods with little added salt and, at the same time, consuming potassium-rich foods such as fruits and vegetables.

The Dietary Reference Intakes (IOM, 2005a) recommend limiting the sodium intake according to age for children and adolescents up to age 18. The higher number in each age category reflects the Upper Level, the maximum level that is likely to pose no risk of adverse effect.

Age (years)	Daily Sodium Intake Range (mg)
2 to 3	1,000 to 1,500
4 to 8	1,200 to 1,900
9 to 13	1,500 to 2,200
14 to 18	1,500 to 2,300

In 2006 the American Medical Association, recognizing the long-term adverse health effects of excess sodium in the diet, recommended that the Food and Drug Administration (FDA) limit the amount of sodium that may be added to commercial foods.

Nonnutritive Food Components

Nonnutritive Sweeteners

Nonnutritive sweeteners, which include aspartame, sucralose, acesulfame-K, neotame, sugar alcohols, and saccharin, are usually consumed in coffee, tea, diet soft drinks, and some low-calorie food items. The goal of inclusion of nonnutritive sweeteners in beverages and foods is to provide a desirable sweet taste without additional calories. In considering nonnutritive sweeteners in competitive foods and beverages for school-age children, four related topics were evaluated: safety of nonnutritive sweeteners for children; effect of intake of foods and beverages containing nonnutritive sweeteners on intake of other foods and beverages to be encouraged (fruits, vegetables, whole grains, and nonfat or low-fat dairy products); efficacy of intake of foods and beverages containing nonnutritive sweeteners in contributing to maintenance of a healthy weight in children; and choice (see Chapter 3 for discussion).

Safety The FDA sets a safety standard for foods or food additives, regulated by the Federal Food, Drug, and Cosmetic Act, of "a reasonable certainty of no harm." The Food Additives Amendment (1958) to the Federal Food, Drug, and Cosmetic Act requires FDA approval for use of an additive prior to its inclusion in a food and requires the manufacturer to prove the additive's safety for the way it will be used. The process of determining whether a food additive such as a nonnutritive sweetener is safe is initiated with a Food Additive Petition, submitted by a manufacturer to the FDA for approval. For foods or food additives that are Generally Recognized as Safe (GRAS), the notifier (manufacturer) makes the safety determination and the FDA reviews the notification for approval.

The FDA has reviewed numerous safety studies on nonnutritive sweeteners and has not, to date, found a safety risk associated with their use (FDA, 2006a). Table 2-1 compares four nonnutritive sweeteners that are or have been in common use in the United States and their current approval status.

The American Dietetic Association concluded (ADA, 2004), in a position paper, that there is no clear evidence that nonnutritive sweeteners, when consumed in a diet concordant with the DGA (ADA, 2004), are harmful to health. A variety of noncaloric sweeteners is now on the market (see Table 2-1), and thus the exposure to any single sweetener may be diluted.

There is a paucity of evidence on long-term health effects in humans from nonnutritive sweeteners, particularly resulting from exposure initiated in childhood. Butchko and Stargel (2001) reviewed several published reports assessing the safety of aspartame. Their review included anecdotal reports of adverse health effects (headache, seizures, or allergic-type reactions); it concluded that these effects were "generally mild and common among consumers" and that there was no evidence for a unique or consistent pattern of symptoms that could be associated with aspartame consumption. Lim et al. (2006) prospectively evaluated the hematopoietic and brain carcinogenic potential of aspartame in adult men and women and concluded that their findings did not support an increased risk for cancer.

TABLE 2-1 Comparison of Nonnutritive Sweeteners

Nonnutritive Sweetener	Characteristics	Approval Status	Labeling Requirements
Aspartame	200× sweeter than sugar; contains phenylalanine, a potential harm for individuals with phenylketonuria	Approved	Must state that the product contains phenylalanine
Acesulfame-K	130× sweeter than sugar; cannot be metabolized so contributes no calories	Approved	None
Saccharin	300× sweeter than sugar; safety concerns about carcinogenicity in rodent models	Approved	Must state that use of the product may be hazardous to health
Cyclamate	Safety concerns about potential carcinogenicity	Banned	None

Weihrauch and Diehl (2004) reviewed the literature for human epidemiological studies on the health effects from exposure to a range of nonnutritive sweeteners (saccharin, cyclamate, aspartame, acesulfame-K, sucralose, alitame, and neotame) from foods and beverages. They found that assessing the carcinogenic potential of a single sweetener from dietary exposure was not feasible, but that the overall carcinogenic risk from nonnutritive sweeteners was negligible. Renwick (1990) reviewed toxicity reports and magnitude of safety factor for acesulfame-K, aspartame, cyclamate, and saccharin. Acceptable daily intake levels were reviewed and shown to be well below a toxic threshold for acesulfame-K, aspartame, and saccharin. The review reported that cyclamate was banned based on dose-response evidence at the upper dose intake level but the results were not reproducible in subsequent independent studies.

There is only one known large-scale study (Soffritti et al, 2005) to have tested aspartame in an animal model, from 8 weeks of age until natural death, at varying doses (ranging from 0 to 100,000 ppm) that include levels comparable to human exposure through foods and beverages. The authors concluded that administration of aspartame, even at low doses, caused an increase in incidence of malignant tumors of both epithelial and mesenchymal origin.

The data from the study were reviewed by the European Food Safety Authority (EFSA, 2006) and the Committee on Carcinogenicity of Chemicals in Food, Consumer Products, and the Environment (COC) of the UK Food Standards Agency. Both EFSA and the COC concluded that the study was flawed based on a number of errors identified by the panels. For example, the report of increased numbers of lymphomas and leukemias may have been related to the presence of chronic inflammatory disease in the lungs of rats, but the investigators failed to test for mycoplasma (a causative agent) in the animal colony. The reported tumors of the renal pelvis were found to be likely related to the treatment because high doses of chemical irritants are known to cause calcium imbalances in the rat, leading to renal tumors. Neither was a dose-response relationship between aspartame intake and tumor incidence established. Another reported flaw was that all the malignant tumor incidences and all tumor-bearing animals were aggregated for statistical purposes, and the reviewers found that the aggregated data were not sufficient to demonstrate the carcinogenic potential of aspartame.

In a rebuttal statement, Soffritti (2006) responded to the criticism that lymphoma and leukemia tumors were related to underlying lung disease, and that such diseases are common when animals are taken to the point of natural death as they were in his study. The author also pointed out that, if an infection were present in the colony, it would have affected males and females equally. The other criticisms to the study were not addressed in the rebuttal statement. To date the findings of the study have not been replicated and published.

Displacement of foods to be encouraged Analyses from national food intake surveys show a trend of increasing intake of soft drinks and decreasing intake of milk and 100-percent juice drinks (Lytle et al., 2000; Nielsen and Popkin, 2004). Studies of caloric soft-drink consumption among school-age children and adolescents also show an association between increased consumption of sweetened beverages and milk displacement (Harnack et al., 1999; Marshall et al., 2005; Storey et al., 2004).

Blum et al. (2005) found a significantly increased intake of both diet soda and sugar-sweetened beverages (100-percent juice and sugar-sweetened soda) and decrease in milk consumption in children over a 2-year period using 24-hour diet recall. Bowman (2002) examined trends in beverage consumption from the 1994–1996 CSFII and found an increasing trend in consumption of beverages that included sugar-sweetened and diet sodas, 100-percent fruit juice, and fruit drinks, and a decreasing trend in milk consumption. The study also found that milk drinkers who did not drink sodas drank more milk than those who drank sodas. A systematic review and meta-analysis of soft-drink consumption and nutrition outcomes found that soft drink (all types) consumption was correlated with decreased milk consumption and decreased calcium intake, although the effect sizes were small (Vartanian et al., 2007). This analysis also related soft drink consumption to decreased intakes of fruit and fiber.

The American Academy of Pediatrics Policy Statement on Soft Drinks in Schools states that soft drink consumption displaces milk consumption, but does not distinguish between displacement by sugar- or nonnutritive-sweetened beverages (AAP, 2004c). The 2005 Dietary Guidelines Advisory Committee (DGAC) did not review evidence about nonnutritive-sweetened foods and beverages in the diets of Americans.

Efficacy of nonnutritive sweeteners Evidence that using nonnutritive-sweetened beverages is effective in promoting weight loss in controlled settings compared with nonnutritive-sweetened foods is inconclusive. Porikos et al. (1977) studied eight obese men and women in a metabolic ward to determine if "covert" substitution (subjects were unaware of the change) of sucrose-containing foods with aspartame could dilute caloric intake. The results showed that obese individuals reduced caloric intake and could maintain body weight with covert substitution of aspartame for sucrose in the diet. A follow-up study (Porikos et al., 1982) used a similar protocol where aspartame was substituted covertly midway through the study. The results showed an initial stabilization of subjects' food intake, followed by an increased intake to compensate for 40 percent of the missing calories.

Food intake then stabilized at 85 percent of baseline and remained at that level until the end of the study. The replacement of sucrose by aspartame in this study showed a tendency to curb weight gain.

Tordoff and Alleva (1990) examined whether nonnutritive-sweetened soft drinks were effective in controlling long-term food intake and body weight among 28 nonobese adult men and women. Individuals who consumed aspartame in soft drinks decreased caloric intake by 7 percent and significantly reduced body weight compared to those who consumed high-fructose corn syrup in soft drinks who increased caloric intake by 13 percent and significantly increased body weight. Foltin et al. (1990) also found that complete energy compensation occurred among adult men who consumed reduced-calorie meals in which the carbohydrate content was reduced by replacing sugar with aspartame.

Rogers and Blundell (1989) found that users of saccharin-sweetened yogurt compensated for the eliminated calories by increasing caloric intake in a subsequent meal. Blackburn et al. (1997), however, found that obese women consuming aspartame-sweetened foods and beverages lost significantly more weight than control subjects (no aspartame) in a multidisciplinary weight loss program that included diet and exercise advice. The study did not address the effect of aspartame-sweetened beverages compared to aspartame-sweetened foods on weight loss.

Raben et al. (2002) investigated the long-term effect of substituting additional foods and beverages with nonnutritive sweetener for those sweetened with sucrose in diets of overweight adults. In contrast to the above-described studies, those subjects who consumed additional foods and beverages containing nonnutritive sweeteners in place of sucrose did not compensate for the lost sucrose calories. The control subjects who consumed additional foods sweetened with sucrose increased their energy intake, body weight and fatness, and blood pressure.

James et al. (2004), in a randomized controlled trial of a 12-month focused education intervention, assessed the effect of reducing consumption of carbonated beverages to prevent weight gain in children aged 7–11 years. The study found a modest reduction in the number of carbonated beverages consumed among subjects in the intervention group compared to controls, and it was associated with a reduction in the number of obese children and those at risk of obesity.

Ebbeling et al. (2006) conducted a pilot study to examine the effect of decreasing intake of sugar-sweetened beverages on body weight in adolescent males and females. The intervention used was replacement of sugar-sweetened beverages with noncaloric beverages for 25 weeks. The study found that decreased consumption of sugar-sweetened beverages had a net effect of decreasing body weight over baseline BMI and the effect was greater among the subjects who consumed more sugar-sweetened beverages at baseline. The 2005 DGAC did not review evidence about nonnutritive sweeteners and there is no recommendation in the DGA about a role for nonnutritive-sweetened beverages (or foods) in the diets of Americans.

Caffeine

Caffeine and related substances (theobromine and theophylline), collectively referred to as methylxanthines, are plant-derived alkaloid compounds that have central nervous system stimulating activity. The primary food and beverage sources are coffee, tea, kola nuts, and chocolate. Examples of caffeine levels in foods and beverages are shown in Table 2-2.

Caffeine-containing beverages (coffee, tea, soft drinks, and "energy drinks") are readily available to consumers. A recent USDA survey of more than 15,000 subjects found that 87 percent of the study population consumed food and beverages that contained caffeine (Frary et al., 2005). The overall average intake noted in this study was 193 mg per day of caffeine, or 1.2 mg caffeine per kg of body weight per day. Among children, the study found caffeine consumption in all age groups: 76 percent of those aged 2–5 years consumed an average of 16 mg/day or 0.4 mg/kg body weight; among those aged 6–11 years, 86 percent consumed an average of 26 mg/day or 0.4 mg/kg body weight. Among males and females aged 12–17 years, 91 percent and 88 percent respectively consumed an average of 80 and 59 mg/day, or 0.5 mg/kg body weight.

Small amounts of caffeine can have a transient positive effect on alertness or ability to concentrate (Dixit et al., 2006; Griffiths and Chausmer,

TABLE 2-2 Average Caffeine Levels in Selected Foods and Beverages

	Serving Size (oz)	Caffeine Content (mg)
Brewed coffee	8	95
Starbucks Frappuccino™ Mocha	9.5	72
Decaffeinated coffee	8	2
Brewed tea	8	47
Iced tea	8	5–11
Coca Cola™ Classic	12	30
Mountain Dew™	12	45
Other non-cola soft drinks	12	0–36
Red Bull™	8.3	67
Hot cocoa	8	5
Chocolate milk	8	5
Chocolate bar	1.75	9

SOURCES: McCusker et al., 2006; USDA/ARS, 2006.

2000). Kenemans and Lorist (1995) found that a single dose of caffeine increased cortical activation, rate of accumulation of information, and speed and accuracy of target selections in male and female undergraduate students (aged 19–29 years) who regularly consumed caffeine, compared to those who did not regularly consume. Similar effects have been found in children (Hughes and Hale, 1998; Leviton, 1992; Rapoport et al., 1981), although the benefit appears to diminish with habitual use (Heatherley et al., 2006). In addition, recent epidemiological evidence supports potential health benefits of caffeine in adults for reducing risk for certain chronic diseases such as colorectal cancer and T2D (Popkin et al., 2006). However, these associations are not well established, and their relevance to caffeine consumption in children is not known.

Findings from studies addressing adverse health effects from caffeine consumption by adults are inconclusive (Higdon and Frei, 2006). Studies on caffeine consumption do not demonstrate a significant association between caffeine intake and adverse effects on reproduction, teratogenesis, tumori-genesis, or myocardial infarction (Abbott, 1986; Curatolo and Robertson, 1983). Studies also have been conducted on other potential adverse health effects including hypertension, fluid homeostasis, cognitive effects, and physical dependence.

Hypertension Nonusers of caffeine may experience an increase in blood pressure when administered an acute dose of caffeine, although the evidence is inconclusive (Green and Suls, 1996; Myers, 2004; Umemura et al., 2006; Winkelmayer et al., 2005).

Fluid homeostasis Some investigators have reported that caffeine increases fluid loss through urination in a dose-dependent manner in healthy adult males (Nussberger et al., 1990; Passmore et al., 1987). Other studies found no association between consumption of caffeine-containing beverages and increased production of urine compared to consuming non-caffeinated beverages by healthy adult male subjects (Dorfman and Jarvik, 1970; Grandjean et al., 2000). Risk for dehydration, however, may increase in situations of extremely hot or cold environments (IOM, 1993, 1996).

Cognitive effects Administration of high doses of caffeine to nonusers and infrequent users may have an adverse effect on short-term recall. Terry and Phifer (1986) found that college students given a 100 mg dose of caffeine prior to a test of short-term recall were not able to recall as many words as control subjects. Erikson et al. (1985) found that among female students, caffeine inhibited recall when word lists were presented at a slow rate, but not at a fast rate. Caffeine had no effect on recall among male subjects. In a double-blind study of young adults, Loke (1988) found no significant effect of caffeine on cognitive, learning, and memory performance, although it did increase subjective ratings for mood.

Physical dependence Continual administration does not change the physiological effect of caffeine, but it frequently leads to tolerance to and physical dependence on caffeine (Griffiths and Chausmer, 2000; Griffiths and Woodson, 1988; James, 1997). Tolerance to a substance can be described as the reduced effectiveness of the substance as a result of regular administration over time (Dews et al., 2002). Discontinuation of a tolerated substance leads to symptoms of withdrawal. Although there is no universally accepted definition for dependence, it has been described as being present during regular administration of a substance if discontinuation precipitates symptoms of withdrawal (O'Brien, 1995). Abrupt removal of caffeine from regular users has been shown to be accompanied by withdrawal symptoms such as headache, drowsiness, irritability, and fatigue (Lader, 1999; Reeves et al., 1995).

Few studies have been done examining dependence on caffeine among school-age children. Oberstar et al. (2002) described caffeine dependence after a 1-year follow-up study of daily use in adolescents. In this study, dependence in adolescents was marked by symptoms of withdrawal similar to those found in adults. Bernstein et al. (2002) characterized symptoms of dependence in a small group of adolescents. Forty-two percent of daily caffeine users reported tolerance and 78 percent described symptoms of withdrawal following reduced intake or cessation.

In 1984, Rapoport et al. conducted a controlled, double-blind caffeine challenge among elementary school-age children who reported either "high" (500 mg/day) or "low" previous daily use of caffeine. After a 2-week period during which children received 5 mg/kg/day, parents of previously low-using children reported that their children were restless, more emotional, and less attentive while receiving caffeine. Parents of previously high users reported that their children had no emotional changes from receiving caffeine, but higher anxiety when they did not receive it.

Baer (1987) investigated the effects of small doses of caffeine (1.6–2.5 mg/kg body weight) on motor activity outcomes in kindergarten children. This study found small and inconsistent effects on off-task and gross motor activity. Leonard et al. (1987) reviewed existing studies for effects of caffeine on adults, fetuses, and animal models and concluded that moderate caffeine consumption probably has no long-term effect on physiological measures such as sleep pattern or mood. Caffeine consumption was found to induce transient changes that included altered mood and sleep patterns when administered to nonusers.

Taken together, the evidence for adverse effects of caffeine use in adults suggests that the greatest risk appears to be for symptoms of physical dependence and withdrawal, such as sleeplessness and irritability. These effects may be similar in children.

Consumption Patterns Among School-Age Children and Adolescents

Fruit and Vegetable Consumption

Diets rich in fruits and vegetables are associated with reduced risk for cardiovascular disease, T2D, certain types of cancer, overweight, and obesity (DHHS, 2000; DHHS/USDA, 2005; Lin and Morrison, 2002). Fruits and vegetables can also be good sources of several nutrients of concern in children's diets. Fisher et al. (2002) found that fruit and vegetable consumption among girls was positively related to micronutrient intake, and negatively associated with fat intake. On average, fruits and vegetables are low in energy density and fat, and high in fiber and other nutrients. Thus incorporating fruits and vegetables into the diet can promote satiety and decrease energy intake (Rolls et al., 2004). For a reference intake of 2,000 calories, two cups of fruits and 2.5 cups of vegetables per day are recommended with amounts adjusting depending on caloric intake level. For school-age children and adolescents, this would result in a range of 2.5 to 6.5 cups (5 to 13 servings) of fruits and vegetables each day for the 1,200 to 3,200 calorie-based diets for these ages (DHHS/USDA, 2005). The DGAC recommends that "no more than one-third of the total recommended fruit group intakes come from fruit juice with the rest coming from whole fruit" (DHHS/USDA, 2004).

National dietary intake data based on 24-hour recalls from the CSFII indicate that only 25 percent of school-age children and adolescents aged 6–19 years had two or more servings of fruits on the day of the survey. Only 36 percent of same-age school children and adolescents consumed three or more servings of vegetables. Moreover, fried potatoes accounted for one-third (32 percent) of the reported vegetable servings (DHHS, 2000). More than one-third of the vegetables in the U.S. food supply consisted of iceberg lettuce, frozen potatoes (mainly french fries), and potato chips (Putnam et al., 2002). Only 6 percent of school-age children and adolescents consumed one-third or more servings from dark green or deep yellow vegetables on a daily basis (DHHS, 2000).

Whole-Grain Consumption

Whole-grain foods, valuable sources of nutrients that include fiber, B vitamins, vitamin E, selenium, zinc, copper, and magnesium, consist of the entire grain seed, usually called the kernel. The process of refining grains for food typically removes most of the bran and some of the germ, resulting in loss of dietary fiber, vitamins, and minerals. Altered kernels, such as those cracked, crushed, or flaked, must retain the same relative proportions of bran, germ, and endosperm as the original grain to be called a whole grain (DHHS/USDA, 2005).

Whole grains also contain phytochemicals and phenolic compounds that play important roles in disease prevention (Slavin et al., 2001). Epidemiological studies link whole-grain consumption to better health and reduced risk for certain cancers, CHD, and T2D, and consumption possibly improves glucose response, increases insulin sensitivity, and improves weight management (DHHS, 2000; DHHS/USDA, 2005).

The DGA (DHHS/USDA, 2005) recommends that school-age children eat at least three daily servings, or half their daily grain intake, as whole grains. Dietary studies indicate that consumption of whole grains is far less than the recommended intake in children, with an average intake of no more than one serving per day (less than 10 percent of Americans consume three servings per day).

In a study of whole-grain consumption by U.S. children using data from the 1994–1996 CSFII, the average whole-grain intake for children aged 6–11 years was 0.9 servings per day; for adolescents it was one serving per day. The proportion of children and adolescents consuming an average of two or more servings of whole grains daily was only 15 percent (Harnack et al., 2003). Ready-to-eat cereals, corn or tortilla chips, and yeast breads were the major sources of whole grains among children and adolescents aged 6–18 years (30, 24, and 17 percent, respectively). Children from low-income households consumed fewer whole grains than those from higher-income households (Harnack et al., 2003).

Barriers to increasing whole-grain consumption include taste perceptions, texture, preparation time, limited availability (whole grains are not as widely available at schools as refined grains), lack of understanding of health benefits, and difficulty in identifying whole-grain foods. Although the FDA has provided guidance on what constitutes a whole grain, consumers are often confused when making decisions about these products at point of purchase or consumption.

The DGA (DHHS/USDA, 2005) recommends consumption of at least 3 ounce-equivalents of whole grains each day to help reduce the risk of several chronic diseases and possibly to help maintain weight. The guidelines also suggest that children increase the amount of whole grains in their diets as they grow, and that, at all calorie levels, all age groups should consume at least half their grains as whole grains to achieve fiber recommendations. The average intake of whole grains is currently less than one serving per day, with less than 10 percent of Americans consuming three servings per day (Cleveland et al., 2000). Grains are most commonly consumed in the form of bread, a standard slice (one ounce-equivalent) contains 16 grams of

---

BOX 2-2
Food and Drug Administration Criteria for Whole Grains

Definition of Whole Grain

The Food and Drug Administration defines whole grains as "cereal grains that consist of the intact, ground, cracked or flaked caryopsis, whose principal anatomical components—the starchy endosperm, germ, and bran—are present in the same relative proportions as they exist in the intact caryopsis."

Whole-Grains Health Claim

"Diets rich in whole grain foods and other plant foods and low in total fat, saturated fat, and cholesterol may help reduce the risk of heart disease and certain cancers."

---

flour. Three ounce-equivalent servings of whole-grain bread would therefore provide 48 grams of whole grains per day. At present, no single mechanism can easily determine what constitutes whole-grain products. However, a number of regulations and guidance documents address whole grains.[2]

FDA guidance On February 17, 2006, the FDA published draft guidance on "Whole Grain Label Statements." The FDA included a definition for what constitutes a whole grain (see Box 2-2). FDA guidance also includes examples of which foods would be considered whole grains and which would not. The FDA is in the process of finalizing this guidance (FDA, 2006b).

FDA whole-grain health claim The FDA requires that any food product that carries the whole-grain health claim must by regulation contain 51 percent or more whole-grain ingredients by weight per reference amount and be low in fat (Box 2-2). This appears to be a more straightforward way of identifying whole-grain products; however, not all products that are rich in whole grains currently display the claim.

USDA standards of identity The only whole-grain bakery products that have Standards of Identity are "whole-wheat bread," "whole-wheat rolls," and "whole-wheat buns." The standard requires that these prod-

---

[2]Comparable ounce-equivalents of other grain-based foods include 5 whole wheat crackers, ½ "mini" bagel, and 1 cup flakes or rounds cereal (SOURCE: http://www.mypyramid.gov/pyramid/grains_counts_print.html).

ucts be made from "whole-wheat flour, bromated whole- wheat flour, or a combination of the two," and any product labeled "whole-wheat bread," "whole-wheat rolls," or "whole-wheat buns" must be made only from whole-wheat flours. The only whole-grain "macaroni products" that have Standards of Identity are "whole-wheat macaroni," "whole-wheat spaghetti," and "whole-wheat vermicelli" (21 CFR Part 136.180; 21 CFR Part 139.138) (FDA, 2006b). A number of whole-grain cereal flours and related products also have a Standard of Identity; however, given the proliferation of whole-grain products on the market, there are many that do not fall into the Standards of Identity categories, but are still good choices to increase whole-grain intake.

HealthierUS School Challenge: Whole-grains resource One of the most comprehensive resources to date is that provided by USDA as part of the HealthierUS School Challenge. The resource was developed as a guide to whole grains for school food authorities interested in applying for the Silver or Gold awards of the HealthierUS School Challenge (SOURCE: http://www.fns.usda.gov/tn/HealthierUS/silvergoldtn.html). This resource draws from the existing regulations and guidance described above (USDA's Standards of Identity and FDA's guidance and health claims) and provides school foodservice operatives with specific ways to determine the whole-grain contribution of a food product.

Whole Grains Council stamp The most common private-sector resource is provided by the Whole Grains Council. In an effort to help Americans more easily identify whole-grain products in the marketplace, the Council developed a pair of symbols to appear on whole-grain products (Figure 2-2). One stamp symbol indicates that a product contains a full 16 grams of whole grain per serving; the other indicates that a product contains 8 grams, qualifying it as ½-serving of whole-grain serving. This is a voluntary resource and may not be available for all eligible foods.

Consumption of Calcium-Rich Foods

Osteoporosis may be considered a pediatric disease manifesting itself in later life, and therefore dietary intake of calcium-rich foods and beverages is important for school-age children. Adequate calcium intake during childhood and adolescence is necessary for the attainment of optimal peak bone mass, which may be important in reducing the risk of osteoporosis and fractures later in life (Greer and Krebs, 2006).

Milk and milk products provide more than 70 percent of the calcium consumed by Americans (DHHS/USDA, 2005). Nondairy sources of calcium include dark green leafy vegetables, tofu set with calcium salts,

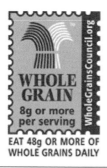

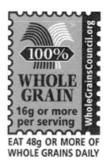

Whole Grain Stamp	100% Whole Grain Stamp
For products providing a half-serving or more of whole grain. Contains at least 8g whole grain per serving. *8g = One-half MyPyramid serving*	For products in which all of the grain is whole grain. Contains at least 16g whole grain per serving. *16g = One MyPyramid serving*

FIGURE 2-2 Identification of qualifying whole-grain products: the Whole Grain Stamps.™
SOURCE: Reprinted, with permission, from Oldways Preservation Trust and the Whole Grains Council (http://www.oldwayspt.org and http://www.wholegrains-council.org). Whole Grain Stamps are a trademark of Oldways Preservation Trust and the Whole Grains Council.

tortillas made from lime-processed corn, and calcium-fortified foods and beverages. Low intakes of calcium in children and adolescents may be related to the displacement of milk intake by soft drinks and juice drinks (Greer and Krebs, 2006; Harnack et al., 1999). Soft-drink consumption peaks in adolescence and milk intake is at its lowest level (Greer and Krebs, 2006).

National dietary survey data consistently show that most children older than 8 years do not consume the recommended amounts of calcium. National CSFII data indicated that only 19 percent of females and 52 percent of males 9–19 years of age met calcium recommendations (1,300 mg calcium/day) (DHHS, 2000). Only 10 percent of adolescent females achieve the recommended adequate dietary intake of calcium (Greer and

Krebs, 2006). There are dairy products, including flavored low-fat and nonfat milks and yogurts, that are popular among school-age children and can make a positive contribution to bone health. Johnson et al. (2002) demonstrated a positive association between flavored-milk consumption and calcium intake among children and adolescents aged 5–17 years. They also found there was no association between consumption of flavored milk and percentage of energy from saturated fat.

Consumption of Added Sugars

Added sugars are sugar or syrup or both added to foods or beverages during processing or preparation. Major sources of added sugars include soft drinks, cakes, cookies, pies, fruit drinks, candy, dairy products, and desserts. These differ from naturally occurring sugars such as fructose in fruits or lactose in milk (IOM, 2002/2005).

Children and adolescents tend to have diets high in added sugars (Briefel and Johnson, 2004). Analysis of the CSFII data (1994–1996) found that added sugars contributed 20 percent of total daily calories in school-age children's diets or about 25 teaspoons per day (Gleason and Suitor, 2001a). Absolute intake of added sugars ranged from 19 teaspoons per day for girls ages 6–8 years to 36 teaspoons per day (3/4 cup) for males aged 14–18 years.

There are no DRI upper reference levels for total or added sugars because there was insufficient evidence to set them (IOM, 2002/2005). However, a maximal intake of 25 percent or less of energy from added sugars was recommended. The Joint World Health Organization/Food and Agriculture Organization of the United Nations Expert Consultation report, *Diet, Nutrition, and the Prevention of Chronic Diseases* (WHO, 2003) recommended that free sugars (equivalent to added sugars) constitute less than 10 percent of total energy in the diet because added sugars provide significant energy without specific nutrients. The DGA (DHHS/USDA, 2005) recommends choosing and preparing foods and beverages with as little as possible added sugars or caloric sweeteners.

Many foods and beverages contain high amounts of added sugars. Flavored yogurts contain about 23–27 grams of added sugars, comprising about 46–48 percent of calories. Most flavored milk contains about 15–16 grams of added sugars, comprising about 35–40 percent of calories. Consumption data from the 1994–1996 and 1998 CSFII on the intake of added sugars show that, for children aged 6–17 years who provided two full days of dietary data, sweetened dairy products were positively associated with calcium intake. Consumption of presweetened cereals was also shown to increase the likelihood of children meeting recommended intake levels for calcium, folate, and iron. Other sources of added sugars, including sweetened baked products and other sweetened prepared grain-based foods, sweets, and sweetened beverages, were associated with a decreased likelihood for meeting recommended intake levels (Frary et al., 2004). Responding to concerns about added sugars while supporting the intake of calcium in milk, the New York State Education Department set a limit of 10 grams of added sugars per 8-ounce serving of nonfat milk sold in schools.

The Nutrition Facts panel on foods and beverages states the amount of total sugars, but does not distinguish between naturally occurring and added sugars. Thus, relying on the current Nutrition Facts panel, it is not possible to determine the amount of added sugar in an item. States and school districts that set limits on added sugars often use the proxy of "percent sugar by weight" and use the total sugar figure on the Nutrition Facts panel to calculate sugar by weight. One standard that has been applied broadly in setting limits on added sugars is "35 percent total sugar by weight" where the total grams of sugar are compared to the total gram weight of the product. However, a criterion based on weight unfairly favors foods higher in moisture content at the expense of drier foods that may be rich in a variety of nutrients (e.g., cereals and granola bars). A standard based on calories, such as "35 percent of calories as total sugar" is still a realistic calculation to do and would allow for a greater variety of products—especially ones that are less moist in nature—to be provided. A measure based on total calories instead of weight is a reasonable option until analytical methods and labeling regulations are established to measure and label the added sugars content of foods and beverages.

Consumption of Sugar-Sweetened Beverages

Although there are naturally occurring sugars in many foods and beverages (milk, fruits, some vegetables), there are many beverages popular with school-age children and adolescents that are composed of high levels of simple sugars, and little other nutrient value. These beverages are a source of concern because their consumption may displace intake of high nutrient-dense beverages such as milk (Blum et al., 2005; Hanson et al., 2005; Rajeshwari et al., 2005; Yen and Lin, 2002).

Fisher et al. (2004) conducted a longitudinal study that examined whether beverage choice, in the context of mother–daughter beverage choices, correlated with calcium intake and bone mineral content in school-age children. Beverage intake included milk, fruit juice, sweetened beverages, and noncaloric beverage and was assessed by 24-hour dietary recall. Intakes were recorded over a course of five years. Milk selection remained relatively constant over the course of the study, while juice intake decreased, and sweetened and noncaloric-beverages intake increased with age. The subjects' intake of non-caloric beverages remained low in absolute amounts, compared to milk and sweetened-beverage intake. Milk intake was found to decrease relative to increased intake of sweetened beverages by age, over time. The study concluded that calcium intake in girls, aged 5–9 years, reflected the relative intake of milk and sweetened beverages in their diet.

Whiting et al. (2001) conducted a longitudinal study to examine whether the amount and type of beverage consumed by adolescent boys and girls correlated with bone mineral content. Beverage and dietary intake data were collected by 24-hour recall over a six-year period. This study found a negative correlation between consumption of nutrient-poor beverages and total body bone mineral content during the 2 years around the age of peak bone mineral accrual in girls. This correlation did not hold up for boys. The authors concluded that milk consumption decreased with increased consumption of nutrient-poor beverages, but their data did not support a relationship between carbonated beverage consumption and bone health (e.g., bone-retarding chemicals in cola drinks). Reduced bone mineral accrual was significantly correlated with milk displacement by nutrient-poor beverages among girls only.

Blum et al. (2005) reviewed existing longitudinal data and found shifts in beverage consumption correlated with increased BMI, but concluded that additional longitudinal data were needed to show an association between substituting low-nutrient-dense beverages for milk and increased BMI in school-age children.

Adolescents, who have the highest intake of added sugars, obtain about 40 percent of their added sugar intake from soft drinks (Briefel and Johnson, 2004). In general, adolescents drink more soft drinks than milk or fruit juices (Briefel and Johnson, 2004). Depending on the study, Popkin et al. (2006) noted that the average calorie intake for all Americans aged 2 and older has increased by 150–300 calories per day over the past 20–30 years. About 50 percent of this increase is contributed by the consumption of sugar-sweetened beverages (Popkin et al., 2006). In the 1990s, soft drinks contributed about 4 percent of total energy intake among 6- to 11-year-old children and 8 percent among adolescents.

Increased added sugars intake has been shown to result in increased energy intake for children (Bowman, 1999). For example, adolescents who did not drink soft drinks consumed 1,984 calories per day compared to 2,604 calories per day for adolescents who drank 26 or more fluid ounces of soft drinks per day (Harnack et al., 1999). In addition, consumption of sugar contribution to dental caries (DHHS/USDA, 2004).

Among obese adolescents, soft drinks contributed about 10 percent of total energy intake for males and about 9 percent for females (Troiano et al., 2000). Soft drinks are not the only sugar-sweetened beverages. Others include fruit drinks and sports drinks. As reported by Guthrie and Morton

(2000), the percentage of total intake of added sweeteners contributed by soft drinks and fruit drinks to the diets of children is as follows:

- Children aged 2–5 years: 34 percent
- Children aged 6–11 years: 35 percent
- Females aged 12–17 years: 48 percent
- Males aged 12–17 years: 50 percent

Several primary studies have found a positive link between obesity and soft-drink consumption (James et al., 2004; Ludwig et al., 2001; Mrdjenovic and Levitsky, 2003; Striegel-Moore et al., 2006; Welsh et al., 2005). Pereira (2006) and Bachman et al. (2006) concluded from a review of studies that the findings were inconsistent, and high-quality randomized trials are needed to evaluate the possible association between changes in sweetened beverage intake and risk for obesity. A systematic review of the literature (Malik et al., 2006) examined sugar-sweetened beverages and weight gain and concluded that the weight of epidemiological and experimental evidence indicated that a greater consumption of sugar-sweetened beverages is associated with weight gain and obesity. In general, reducing consumption of sweetened beverages is viewed as an important component of a broad strategy to reduce excess energy intake (Dietz, 2006; Popkin et al., 2006).

Consumption of Fat

The role of fat in the diet is complicated because different types of fatty acids have different effects on health. However, it is clear that children consume too much dietary fat, and too much of the fat is from saturated fatty acids (DHHS, 2000). Troiano et al. (2000) found that only one in four school-age children met the intake guidelines for total fat and saturated fat. Among 9- to 13-year-old males, only 14 percent met the dietary fat recommendation of 30 percent or less of total calories from fat and only 6 percent met the saturated fat recommendation (Gleason and Suitor, 2001a). Data are consistent that diets low in saturated fatty acids are associated with lower risk for and lower rates of CHD (DHHS, 2000).

The DGA recommends that children and adolescents 4–18 years of age consume 25–35 percent of their calories from fat, with most fats coming from polyunsaturated and monounsaturated fatty acids. Less than 10 percent of calories should come from saturated fats and trans fat intake should be kept as low as possible (DHHS/USDA, 2005). For individuals with elevated blood cholesterol levels, the recommended saturated fat intake is less than 7 percent of total calories (DHHS/USDA, 2005).

The trans fats found in hydrogenated oils not only increase low-density lipoprotein (LDL) cholesterol as do saturated fats, but also decrease high-density lipoprotein (HDL) cholesterol. These combined effects result in a larger increase in total cholesterol:HDL cholesterol ratio than is observed for dietary saturated fats (Grundy, 1999).

Population trends show that the U.S. population has decreased total fat intake while increasing its caloric intake (Troiano et al., 2000), and has experienced population-wide weight gain (Ogden et al., 2006). These trends suggest that fat intake is not the only cause of obesity. A low-fat diet will not necessarily lead to weight loss if the total caloric value of the diet exceeds the individual's energy needs.

Nevertheless, fats are calorie dense, and a high fat intake is a major contributor to the high caloric intake of overweight and obese individuals (Prentice, 2001). In addition, diets high in fat tend to contain levels of saturated fats that exceed the DRI (IOM, 2002/2005). Extremely low-fat diets may be low in essential fatty acids and impair absorption of fat-soluble vitamins, but this is rare in healthy children. The primary sources of saturated fats are meats and dairy products. Trans fatty acids are found in many processed snack foods and baked products, although there are trace amounts in animal foods such as milk and meats.

Consumption of Foods of Low Nutrient Density

Nutrient-dense foods are those foods that provide relatively high amounts of vitamins and minerals (micronutrients) and relatively few calories (DHHS/USDA, 2005). Foods of low nutrient density are those that supply calories but no or small amounts of micronutrients. Foods of low nutrient density represent a high contribution to energy and fat intakes. The top ten foods contributing to energy intakes in children aged 2–18 years are milk, bread, cakes/cookies/quick breads/doughnuts, beef, ready-to-eat cereal, soft drinks, cheese, potato chips/corn chips/popcorn, sugars/syrup/jams, and poultry; several of these foods such as soft drinks, chips, cakes, cookies, and pastries, are low-nutrient-dense foods (Subar et al., 1998).

The CSFII 1994–1996 survey found that added sugars and fat contributed 45 percent of total energy intake in school-age children, with sugars contributing 20 percent of total calories and discretionary fat calories 25 percent (Gleason and Suitor, 2001a). In NHANES III, foods of low nutrient density contributed more than 30 percent of total energy intake among school-age children, with sweetened beverages, candy, and desserts providing about 25 percent of total energy intake (Kant, 2003). One-third of school-age children and adolescents reported eating six or more foods of low nutrient density on the day of recall. Mean intakes of vitamins and minerals declined with increasing number of calorie-dense foods consumed (Kant, 2003). Consumption of foods of low nutrient density was related to higher energy consumption but was not associated with BMI.

In general, greater consumption of calorie-dense foods and beverages makes it more difficult to consume sufficient nutrients without gaining weight, especially for those individuals who are inactive (DHHS/USDA, 2005). If nutrient-dense foods are selected exclusively from the various food groups in the amounts recommended, then only a relatively small amount of calories is available to be consumed as added fats or added sugars (DHHS/ USDA, 2005). This is called the discretionary calorie allowance. Calorie needs are variable in children and adolescents and depend on age, rate of growth, level of physical activity, body size and composition, and stage of sexual maturation. The amount of discretionary calories increases as total caloric need increases, and is strongly associated with physical activity level. With increasing physical activity levels, discretionary calories increase. At 1,600, 2,000 and 3,000 total calories per day, the discretionary calorie allowance would be 132, 267, and 512 calories, respectively. For sedentary children and adolescents, the discretionary calorie allowance may only be 150 to 250 calories per day. This small amount of discretionary calories does not allow consumption of many calorie-dense snacks and beverages. For example, a 20-ounce soft drink contains 250 calories. Figure 2-3 illustrates the concept of essential calories (the total energy necessary to meet recommended nutrient intakes) and discretionary calories. As can be seen for inactive children, only small amounts of discretionary calories can be consumed before caloric intake becomes excessive and weight gain results (Gidding et al., 2006). Butte (2006) estimated energy requirements for children based upon reports by the Institute of Medicine (2002/2005) and Food and Agriculture Organization of the United Nations/World Health Organization/United Nations University (2004). These estimates of energy intake recommendations for children 11 years of age and under were lower than the 1985 FAO/WHO recommendations due to decreased total energy expenditure in this age group.

The committee estimated the amount of dietary energy available for discretionary energy consumption as snacks based on daily energy requirements for boys and girls as a function of age and physical activity level (IOM, 2002/2005) Estimating that approximately 25 percent of daily energy intake would be consumed at breakfast, 33 percent at lunch, and 33 percent at dinner would leave approximately 9 percent of total daily energy intake for discretionary calorie consumption. These calculations are also consistent with guidelines of the School Breakfast and National School Lunch Programs. Appendix Tables B-1 and B-2 depict the estimated energy requirements provided in the DRI report (IOM, 2002/2005) for children

64

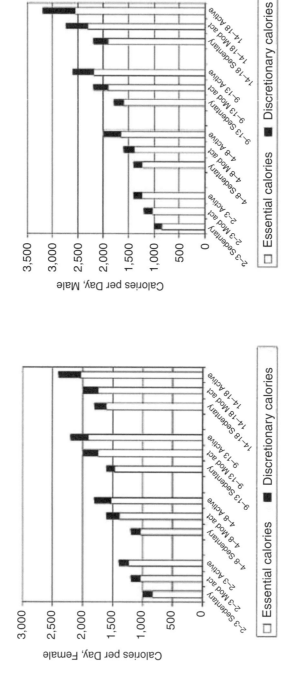

FIGURE 2-3 Essential and discretionary calories by gender, age, and level of activity.
SOURCE: Reprinted, with permission, from *Pediatrics* 117(2):544–559. Copyright 2006 by the American Academy of Pediatrics.

and include an additional four columns that show the number of calories in 9 percent of total daily energy intake allotted as discretionary calories derived from snacks.

Fast Food Consumption

National CSFII (1994–1996, 1998) data using 24-hour diet recalls indicate that on a typical day 33 percent of children aged 9–19 years reported eating foods obtained at fast-food and pizza outlets (excluding the school cafeteria). This included 26 percent of children aged 9–13 years and 39 percent of adolescents aged 14–19 years (Bowman et al., 2004). Fast-food consumption was prevalent in both sexes, all racial/ethnic groups, and all regions of the country. Increased consumption was independently associated with male gender, adolescent age, higher household incomes, non-Hispanic black race/ethnicity, and residence in the South.

Fast-food consumption can have a negative impact on the nutritional quality of the diets of children and adolescents and may increase risk for obesity. CSFII data showed that children who consumed fast food compared with those who did not consumed more total energy (187 calories), total fat, and soft drinks, and less milk, fruits, and non-starchy vegetables (Bowman et al., 2004) compared with those who did not. French et al. (2001) found in a survey with 4,746 adolescents of multiple ethnicities that frequency of fast-food restaurant use was positively associated with total energy, energy from fat, and servings of soft drinks and french fries, and was negatively associated with servings of fruit, vegetables, and milk. A study of 101 girls between the ages of 8–12 at baseline and 11–19 years at follow-up found that the frequency of eating fast food at baseline was positively associated with change in BMI z-score. Girls who ate fast food twice a week or more at baseline had the greater mean increase in BMI z-score compared to those who ate fast food once a week or less (Thompson et al., 2004). These results suggest that fast food consumption can promote a positive energy balance and weight gain.

Meal and Snack Patterns

Another way of examining children's dietary intake is to look at meal and snack patterns. Children and adolescents are more likely to skip breakfast than lunch or dinner. Based on CSFII data from 1994–1996, nearly one in five (19 percent) school-age children ate nothing for breakfast on the day of the survey (i.e., any given day), and one in three (33 percent) consumed foods and beverages that contributed less than 10 percent of their daily recommended energy allowance (Gleason and Suitor, 2001a). The percentage of children and adolescents who skipped breakfast on the day of the survey increased with age: 8 percent of those aged 6–8 years, 14 percent aged 9–13 years, and 31 percent aged 14–18 years. Omitting breakfast was most frequent among adolescent females (14–18 years), with 34 percent not eating breakfast. Among all school-age children and adolescents, breakfast provided an average of 18 percent of total daily energy intake. Breakfast, when consumed, tended to be lower in fat compared to other meals (Gleason and Suitor, 2001a). Breakfast consumption has been shown to be associated with more favorable nutrient intakes and improved dietary quality in children and adolescents (Nicklas et al., 1993; Rampersaud et al., 2005). These studies found that children who eat breakfast are more likely to meet recommended intakes for vitamins and minerals than those who skip breakfast. Barton et al. (2005) found an association with cereal eating and decreased risk for obesity. In this study, however, breakfast eating was not significantly associated with decreased risk for obesity.

The majority of studies, though not all, have shown that breakfast eaters are less likely to be obese (Affenito et al., 2005; Barton et al., 2005; Rampersaud et al., 2005). A recent study examined trends in adolescent obesity from 1971 to 2004 using NHANES data (Miech et al., 2006). Skipping breakfast on the day of the 24-hour dietary survey was significantly associated with being obese. Evidence also suggests that eating breakfast may improve cognitive function related to memory and increase school attendance (Rampersaud et al., 2005).

Not eating lunch is less common than skipping breakfast. Just less than 10 percent of children and adolescents aged 6 to 18 years ate nothing for lunch on the day of the CSFII survey. Lunch provided nearly one-third of the energy for the day (Gleason and Suitor, 2001a). Dinner is frequently consumed by children and adolescents, but not necessarily with their family. In response to the survey question "How many times did all, or most, of your family living in your house eat a meal together?" about 22–32 percent of older children and adolescents reported eating dinner as a family only a few days a week or never (Gillman et al., 2000; Neumark-Sztainer et al., 2003). These studies along with Videon and Manning (2003) suggest that eating meals as a family may influence dietary intake of children. Increasing frequency of family dinner is also associated with consumption of more fruits and vegetables, less fried food and soft drinks, less saturated and trans fat, and more fiber, calcium, vitamins and minerals (Gillman et al., 2000; Neumark-Sztainer et al., 2003).

Most U.S. children consume at least one snack per day (Cross et al., 1994), and snacking prevalence among children has increased since 1977 (Jahns et al., 2001). Data from national surveys show that, on average, school-age children snack about twice daily (Cross et al., 1994; Huang et al., 2004; Jahns et al., 2001), consuming nearly one-quarter of energy intake as snacks (Huang et al., 2004; Jahns et al., 2001).

The energy density of foods is higher for snacks compared to meals (Jahns et al., 2001). Based on the 1994–1996 and 1998 CSFII, children 3–5 years of age ate snacks averaging 146 ± 3 calories, children 6–11 years of age ate snacks averaging 197 ± 5 calories, and adolescents aged 12–19 years ate snacks averaging 274 ± 11 calories (Huang et al., 2004).

Food Choice Behavior

Studies of the effects of children's consumption patterns on parents restricting energy-dense foods suggests that severe restriction of preferred foods of low nutrient value may increase their desire for such foods (Benton, 2004; Fisher and Birch, 1999). Taste perception is likely another important factor in food choices (Drewnowski, 1997). Factors that determine taste preference include genetic background (Birch, 1999; Mennella et al., 2005) and early life exposure (Birch, 1998; Birch and Fisher, 1998; Mennella et al., 2006). Because schools represent only a small part of the daily eating opportunity for children it is not clear whether restriction of energy-dense foods of minimal nutritional value in the school environment will encourage school-age children to consume them.

Studies of students' perceptions of factors influencing food choices suggest that they are open to information about healthful choices and willing to make changes to improve their diets. O'Dea (2003) studied the responses of students aged 7–17 years to suggested strategies to overcome barriers to healthful eating. This study found that children and adolescents were willing to make healthful behavior changes and looked to parents and teachers for support. Neumark-Sztainer et al. (1999) assessed perceptions of factors that affect food choice behaviors among adolescent boys and girls from inner-city schools. From focus group discussions, the study identified a broad range of factors such as hunger, taste appeal, availability, and convenience that influence food choice behavior. The study concluded that knowledge of these factors could be useful in developing ways to make healthful food more appealing to adolescents and encourage healthful behaviors.

SOCIODEMOGRAPHIC FACTORS AFFECTING DIETS IN CHILDHOOD AND ADOLESCENCE

Gender

Gender differences in dietary intakes emerge as children move into adolescence. During childhood, food intakes of girls and boys tend to be similar. Because of increased rates of growth and body size, adolescent males eat larger quantities of food on average than female adolescents, so they are more likely to meet recommended daily intakes for vitamins and minerals. Dietary surveys show adolescent males eat more servings of grains, vegetables (including french fries), dairy, and meat compared to adolescent females (Enns et al., 2003; Gleason and Suitor, 2001a). Adolescent males are also more likely to have diets higher in total fat and saturated fat (Gleason and Suitor, 2001a) and to consume larger amounts of soft drinks (French et al., 2003). As a group, adolescent females are more likely to have lower intakes of vitamins and minerals (Enns et al., 2003; Gleason and Suitor, 2001a; Story et al., 2002b). They are also more likely to skip meals, especially breakfast, than are adolescent males (Gleason and Suitor, 2001a). In fact, dietary data show that adolescent females aged 14–18 years have the poorest diets compared to all other age or gender groups (Gleason and Suitor, 2001a).

Economic Status

Children in low-income families fare less well than children in more affluent families on many health status indicators (DHHS, 2000; FIFCFS, 2005). In 2003, 18 percent of all children up to 17 years of age lived in poverty. The poverty rate was higher for African American (34 percent) and Hispanic (30 percent) children compared to white children (10 percent) (FIFCFS, 2005). About 12.4 million children (16.9 percent) lived in households that were classified as food insecure at times in 2005. Households are classified as food insecure based on reports of difficulty obtaining enough food, reduced dietary quality, and anxiety about food supplies (USDA/ERS, 2006).

Several studies have shown that children in families below the poverty level are less likely than higher-income children to have a healthy diet (Devaney et al., 1995; FIFCFS, 2005; Fox and Cole, 2004; Munoz et al., 1997). Studies of trends in obesity show that patterns between socioeconomic status and overweight are complex, but such associations can be drawn (Melgar-Quinonez and Kaiser, 2004; Ritchie et al., 2003; Sturm, 2005; Wang and Zhang, 2006). In these studies, children and adolescents in low-income families had higher intakes of total and saturated fat and consumed less fruit and dairy products. Low socioeconomic status has been shown to be a strong predictor of low fruit and vegetable intake among adolescents (Neumark-Sztainer et al., 1996). This may be related to financial resources to purchase fruits and vegetables and less access to affordable, quality fruits and vegetables in low-income communities.

Current child poverty rates highlight the importance of the federal child nutrition programs such as the National School Lunch Program (NSLP) and the School Breakfast Program (SBP), which provide a food and nutrition safety net for low-income children to help reduce hunger and improve health. In the 2005–2006 school year, the NSLP provided lunch to 29 million children and adolescents on an average day. Of these, 17 million (59 percent) received a free or reduced-price school lunch (FRAC, 2006).

Race and Ethnicity

National CSFII data for school-age children found that African American and Hispanic children and adolescents were less likely to meet recommendations for limiting total and saturated fat than their white counterparts, and total consumption of milk products and calcium was lowest among African American children and adolescents. White children had the highest intake of added sugars and soft drinks, although African Americans drank more fruit drinks (Gleason and Suitor, 2001a). Other studies have also shown that white children drank more milk than African American children, and that African American girls drank more fruit drinks (Storey et al., 2004; Striegel-Moore et al., 2006).

DIETARY TRENDS OVER TIME AMONG SCHOOL-AGE CHILDREN

Changes over time in school-age children's food consumption (Gidding et al., 2005) include

- increased consumption of foods prepared away from home;
- increased percentage of total calories from snacks;
- increased consumption of calorie-dense foods;
- increased portion sizes of foods;
- increased consumption of sweetened beverage; and
- decreased consumption of milk.

Trends in Dietary and Nutrient Intakes

A recent study examined dietary intake trends among children and adolescents over a 20-year period using data from three USDA national surveys: Nationwide Food Consumption survey 1977–1978; CSFII 1989–1991; and CSFII 1994–1996, 1998 (Enns et al., 2002, 2003). Among children 6 to 11 years old and adolescents 12 to 19 years old, increases in dietary intakes over time were found for soft drinks, total grain products, snack chips, fried potatoes, fruit drinks, and candy (Enns et al., 2002, 2003). The intake of chips, crackers, popcorn, and pretzels roughly tripled from the mid-1970s to the mid-1990s for both children and adolescents. The intake of soft drinks roughly doubled during this same period for children and adolescent females and tripled among adolescent males. In both age groups, decreases were found for total milk intake. Total fat intake and percentage of calories from fat decreased, but this was due in part to increased carbohydrate intake (Enns et al., 2002, 2003). For example, among children, fat intake decreased by 100 calories or less, but carbohydrate intake increased by about 150–200 calories (Sturm, 2005). NHANES trend data from the 1970s to 1999–2000 also found a decrease in dietary fat and percentage of energy from fat and concomitant increases in carbohydrate intake among children and adolescents (Briefel and Johnson, 2004). The CSFII data showed increases in iron and thiamin intake, and decrease in vitamin B12 in children and adolescents (Enns et al., 2002, 2003).

Dietary Changes Among Children

National data indicate that diet adequacy deteriorates as individuals get older; children, especially infants and young children, have diets that are more nutritionally adequate than those of adolescents (Devaney et al., 2005). Lytle et al. (2000), in a longitudinal study of 291 student participants, found that diet quality declines as children move from middle childhood into adolescence; intake of fruits, vegetables, and milk decreases and consumption of soft drinks increases. The study showed that fruit consumption fell by 41 percent between the third and eighth grades and vegetable consumption fell by 25 percent. Additional evidence from a longitudinal study of girls (Mannino et al., 2004) showed that dietary quality declined between 5 and 9 years of age, with a larger proportion of girls at 9 years of age having inadequate intakes of dairy, fruits and vegetables, and several nutrients than they did at an earlier age. Lin et al. (2001) determined that an increase in eating out was a factor in the age-related adolescent decline in diet quality.

Trends in Meal Patterns and Snacking

Breakfast consumption by U.S. children and adolescents has declined over time. For example, between 1965 and 1991, breakfast consumption declined 9 percent in children aged 8 to 10 years and 13 to 20 percent in adolescent males and females. The greatest decline (20 percent) was in adolescent girls (Siega-Riz et al., 1998). The nutritional quality of foods consumed at breakfast has improved since 1965, especially in substitution of lower fat for full-fat milk (Siega-Riz et al., 1998). The introduction of the SBP has increased breakfast consumption among children in low-income areas. The Bogalusa Heart Study found that from 1973 to 1978, there was a marked increase from 8 to 30 percent in the percentage of children who skipped breakfast. When school breakfast service was introduced in the district in 1981, the percentage of children skipping breakfast declined to 12 percent (Nicklas et al., 2004).

Nationally representative data also show that the prevalence of snacking has increased in school-age children and adolescents from 1977 to 1996. The average size of snacks and energy content per snack remained relatively constant during this period; however, the number of snacks eaten per day rose significantly, thus increasing the average daily energy from snacks (Jahns et al., 2001). Nielsen and colleagues (2002) found that CSFII data showed the increase in energy intake occurred predominantly from snacks particularly from 1989 to 1996 among adolescents. Thus the increase in snacking may be contributing to the epidemic of obesity in children and adults (Jahns et al., 2001; Zizza et al., 2001).

Trends in Portion Sizes

Portion sizes have increased steadily over the past 30 years (Nielsen et al., 2002; Young and Nestle, 2002). Data suggest that the trend toward larger portion sizes began in the 1970s, increased sharply in the 1980s, and has continued to increase (Young and Nestle, 2002). Between 1977 and the mid-1990s, food portion sizes for Americans aged 2 years and older increased both inside and outside the home for salty snacks, desserts, soft drinks, fruit drinks, french fries, hamburgers, cheeseburgers, and Mexican-type foods (Nielsen et al., 2002).

Larger portions not only contain more calories, but also encourage people to eat more. A recent controlled laboratory study found that increasing the portion size of all foods resulted in a significant increase in energy intake that was sustained over two days (Rolls et al., 2006). Because portion size affects energy balance, there is a need for greater attention to food portion size and consuming recommended serving sizes, such as those in the DGA.

LIMITATIONS IN RESEARCH ON CHILDREN'S DIETS

Measuring what people eat and drink is one of the most challenging aspects of population-based nutrition research studies. Studies assessing dietary intake patterns; nutrient intakes and nutrition; and health and disease relationships, especially population-based epidemiological studies, rely predominantly on self-reporting using dietary assessment instruments such as 24-hour recalls, diet records, or food frequency questionnaires. Although it is recognized that self-reported dietary intake data reflects underestimates of food intake and, in turn, energy intake, the magnitude of this effect in different populations is not clear. Studies using doubly-labeled water show that underreporting of food intake is pervasive in adults. Underreporting constitutes anywhere from 10 to 45 percent of the total, depending on the age, gender, and weight of the respondents (Johnson, 2000). Underreporting tends to increase in prevalence as children mature, is more common among women than men, and is higher among overweight and obese adults (Johnson, 2000).

Other factors associated with underreporting include perceived social desirability of intake patterns, body image dissatisfaction, dieting, and greater eating restraint (Maurer et al., 2006). Social desirability may influence not only self-reported total energy intake, but also the likelihood of underreporting socially undesirable food intake patterns such as the consumption of high-fat, high-sugar foods and beverages (Maurer et al., 2006). On the other hand, social desirability of healthy foods such as fruits and vegetables can result in overreporting (Maurer et al., 2006).

Misreporting of food intake may result from errors in the estimation of portion sizes, inability or unwillingness to record or remember everything that was eaten, unintentional omission of certain foods or portions, and deliberate misreporting. Engaging in the recording process or anticipating the report of food intake may cause an individual to temporarily change the way he or she eats (Maurer et al., 2006). It is also more difficult to remember what was eaten between meals, which is an issue for children and adolescents who may snack frequently. Dietary intake research on young children also presents special challenges; the child's parent or teacher may be relied on to recall the child's intake, thus introducing a third party and further complicating the assessment process (Goran, 1998).

3

The School Environment

INTRODUCTION

The organizational structure of the schools is an important consideration in formulating recommendations for standards for competitive foods and beverages in schools. U.S. school systems are complex organizations. Internally, they are made up of many different constituencies competing for limited organizational resources. Externally, they must respond to the varied requirements and constraints imposed by federal and state agencies, as well as taxpayers and parents. Decisions governing the availability of competitive foods are interwoven in this complicated structure.

This chapter describes the way in which competitive foods are connected to the complex school environment. Although the committee's primary task was to define nutritional standards based on health considerations and the committee was not charged with developing a detailed implementation plan, the ultimate goal of optimizing the overall school nutrition environment will be determined largely by the extent to which local, state, and federal policymakers anticipate and address a variety of implementation challenges. This chapter identifies these challenges and provides the background for related recommendations in Chapter 5. The chapter first addresses the organization of the U.S. public school system, then provides an operational description of the National School Lunch Program (NSLP) and the School Breakfast Program (SBP). Although foods and beverages offered through these programs are not included in the committee's definition of competitive foods, they set the food-service context within which many competitive foods and beverages are provided.

ORGANIZATION OF PUBLIC SCHOOLS

Federal, State, and Local Governance

The federal role in education is limited to certain issues, such as laws involving civil rights and the rights of disabled and at-risk students. The relevant federal legislation includes Title I of the Elementary and Secondary Education Act of 1965, which includes the No Child Left Behind Act of 2001; Richard Russell National School Lunch Act; Child Nutrition Act of 1966; Title IX of the Education Amendments of 1972, which includes the Individuals with Disabilities Education Act; and the Civil Rights Act of 1964.

The American public school system, providing for nearly 50 million children aged 4 through 19, is primarily the responsibility of individual states; within the states, it is the shared responsibility of multiple partners. Each state's governor can create policy through executive order; the legislature can create policy through the development of law; the chief state school officer makes policy; and the state board of education creates policy through a variety of mechanisms including rule making, regulation, and, in some states, self-executing powers. The chief state school officer and the state board of education, with the assistance of the state department of education, are charged with the task of seeing that all laws and regulations are carried out by the local boards of education.

The chief state school officer may be appointed by the governor or the state board of education, or he or she may be elected by partisan or nonpartisan statewide ballot. Membership on the state board of education may also be either by appointment or by election. In 32 states, the state school board members are appointed by the governor; 10 have elected boards and 8 have other arrangements.

Each state is composed of school districts governed by a local school board. Local school board members are usually elected, although in some states they are appointed. Local school board members make up the largest group of elected officials in the United States, totaling about 95,000 members. These officials bear the responsibility for translating state and federal laws and regulations into workable school district policies, and they have the authority to develop operations of their local schools, as long as those policies are consistent with state and federal laws and regulations.

Professional organizations such as the National Governors Association, the National Conference of State Legislatures, the Council of Chief State

School Officers, the National Association of State Boards of Education, and the National School Boards Association represent their members in policy-setting contexts and offer services and training that help members strengthen state and local leadership in educational policy making. Membership in these organizations also provides school board members access to information concerning new and established federal and state laws.

Educational Funding Sources

Federal funding, determined by Congress during the budget process, accounts for about 7 to 10 percent of most local education budgets. Additional funding mechanisms for the balance are determined by the state legislatures. In some states, the major source of funding is the state government, while in others it is the local school districts. Property taxes are a major source of funding for education, along with sales taxes, utility taxes, lottery revenue, statewide and local levies, and state general fund revenue.

Each state has its own method of determining how monies are levied and collected, and local boards of education generally have the authority to pass local taxes to support the local schools. Local funding also enables school districts to go beyond the minimum requirements of state and federal laws that govern their schools.

Revenue also accrues to many schools from the sale of federally reimbursable meals under the NSLP and SBP, and some states allocate state money to support various school meal programs. In addition, most school districts receive revenue from the sale of compatititive foods and beverages. Data presented later in this chapter suggest that overall revenues from competitive foods and beverages are small in relation to total school budgets—less than 1 percent for most schools. However, these monies often play an important role in school operations because they constitute a significant proportion of funds available for certain activities.

Administration of School Nutrition Programs

The NSLP and SBP are usually administered by the state departments of education, though sometimes state departments of agriculture assume this role. Federal regulations require that participating districts designate a School Food Authority (SFA) to operate the program. The SFA can be determined at the local school level, but this occurs more often at the school-district level.

Districts enter into annual agreements with relevant state departments of education to participate in the federally reimbursable school meals programs. In implementing these programs, districts are required to follow established procedures involving reporting on meals served and claiming reimbursements. The state department of education is responsible for training, technical assistance, and monitoring for these programs.

Local school boards set broad food service policy to be executed by school staff. SFAs plan menus, purchase food, oversee meal preparation and service, and keep records that document claims for reimbursement. SFAs work with principals in setting meal schedules and making other arrangements for meals. Nevertheless, the food service programs are typically administered on a district-wide basis rather than at the school level. Although some states and some school districts pay part of the meal program's costs from nonfood revenue, many SFAs are expected to cover costs from revenues generated. However, for all SFAs, any revenue in excess of costs must be reinvested in the meal programs; under federal regulations, schools cannot make a profit from their federally reimbursable school nutrition programs.

NATIONAL SCHOOL LUNCH AND SCHOOL BREAKFAST PROGRAMS

Created in 1946, the NSLP provides meals in most public schools throughout the country as well as in a substantial number of private schools, and currently provides lunch to about 29 million children daily. Participating children from low-income families receive meals either free or at a reduced price, with the federal government providing subsidies to the schools for meals. Children from families that do not meet the income criteria for these free or reduced-price meals are referred to as full-price participants; however, schools also receive a small subsidy for those meals.

To participate in the program, schools are required to comply with regulations designed to ensure that meals served under the programs are healthful and nutritious. However, there is considerable flexibility permitted for meeting these requirements.

A parallel but formally separate program, the SBP provides breakfast to children at school. Although considerably smaller in participation level than the NSLP, the breakfast program is substantial, serving about 9 million breakfasts on a typical day. Although the program is available to all children, more than 80 percent of participants are from low-income families. After-school snacks can be provided by schools through the NSLP or the Child and Adult Care Food Program.

Although foods and beverages sold as part of the NSLP and SBP are not among the competitive foods and beverages that are the focus of this report, they inform the definition of competitive foods. Furthermore, these two programs provide the school food service context that establishes how competitive foods and beverages are provided. Understanding how the federally reimbursable meal programs work is therefore of great importance to the committee's task.

Regulation of School Meal Programs

The NSLP and SBP are authorized under federal legislation, and related federal regulations are determined by the U.S. Department of Agriculture (USDA), Food and Nutrition Service. State agencies, usually the state department of education, develop state regulations based on federal law and regulations, as well as relevant state legislation regarding the operations of the program, and monitor compliance at the school level. These state agencies serve as intermediaries in the fiscal reimbursement process, consolidating reimbursement requests from within the state and transmitting them to USDA.

Day-to-day operations of the programs, including certifying students' eligibility for subsidies, preparing food, and conducting food service operations, is the responsibility of the SFA, which is usually coincident with school districts. In some instances, a group of school districts may combine to form a single SFA. Some SFAs contract with outside vendors for food preparation or other aspects of operations.

Federal Reimbursement for School Meal Programs

Federal reimbursement to the SFA is set on a per-meal basis, with the level of the subsidies determined largely by federal legislation. Federal law requires that students whose families have incomes below certain levels are not charged for meals. The legislation also sets the maximum price allowable for reduced-price meals (currently 40 cents for lunch and 30 cents for breakfast). Schools with high rates of participation by low-income students receive slightly higher reimbursement rates. SFAs are allowed to set the price of the full-price meals they sell. They also determine which qualifying foods are served, subject to detailed regulations designed to ensure that the meals are nutritious and healthful.

There is no federal requirement that SFA must be cost/revenue neutral on their food service operations. However, many school districts expect food service operations to cover their costs without district subsidies. Many SFAs report that they find themselves squeezed by these local financial expectations on the one hand and the federal regulations on the other. In some instances, SFAs use competitive food and beverage sales, which are subject to fewer regulations and allow more flexibility in SFA decision making, to meet the financial expectations of their districts.

Nutrition Requirements for School Meal Programs

From its inception, the NSLP emphasized the importance of providing nutritious meals. Until the 1990s, this was done by specifying "meal pattern," which required that the meals served included certain generic components, such as milk; a protein source; breads, grains, and cereals; and fruits or vegetables. Detailed regulations and guidelines defined exactly what foods and beverages and what serving sizes met these specifications.

In the early 1990s, the first School Nutrition Dietary Assessment (SNDA-I) (Burghardt et al., 1993) found evidence that, although school meals were generally meeting or exceeding various nutrient requirements, they substantially exceeded the Dietary Guidelines for Americans (DGA) recommended limits for total and saturated fat. These observations, together with other factors, led to a series of legislative actions that changed the nutrition requirements of the program. New regulations specified that fat content conform to federal recommendations. They also encouraged greater attention to sodium, cholesterol, and fiber content, and changed methods for monitoring school meals.

The revised system that emerged allows three ways of satisfying nutrition requirements:

1. Schools develop menus using a computer-assisted, nutrient-based system;
2. Alternatively, schools continue to use a food-based system, which is essentially the same as the previous meal pattern requirements; or
3. Schools use an enhanced food-based pattern that includes additional requirements for grains and vegetables.

The regulations also allow SFAs to provide other alternatives for meeting requirements.

COMPETITIVE FOODS AND BEVERAGES

Definition and Overview

The term "competitive foods" is used in this report to include all foods and beverages that are sold, served, or given to students in the school environment other than meals served through the NSLP, SBP, and After-School Snack and Meal Programs. Competitive foods may be available in à la carte lines, snack bars, student stores, vending machines, or school activities, such as fund-raisers, achievement rewards, classroom parties or snacks, school celebrations, and school meetings. They do not include brown bag lunches. The nutritional value of competitive foods and beverages is largely unregulated by the federal government. Furthermore, availability is usually not overseen by the school food service staff. As a result, competitive foods and beverages reflect a broad range of energy and nutrient content. Some competitive foods and beverages consist of healthful items, such as fruits and vegetables. However, many are snack foods and beverages that are calorie dense, nutrient poor, and contain high levels of fat, sugar, and sodium.

Federal regulation has labeled a subcategory of competitive foods and beverages as Foods of Minimal Nutritional Value (FMNV). USDA defines FMNV as those that provide very low amounts per portion for each of eight specified nutrients: protein, vitamins A and C, niacin, riboflavin, thiamin, calcium, and iron. Included in this category are carbonated soft drinks, chewing gum, water ices, and certain candies made predominantly from sweeteners. Schools participating in the NSLP are prohibited from selling FMNV during meal periods in school cafeterias and other food service areas (GAO, 2005). Schools are also prohibited from designing food service areas in such ways that encourage or facilitate the choice or purchase of FMNV as a ready substitute for, or addition to, federally reimbursable meals.

The federal regulations dealing with FMNV set a minimum standard. This does not preclude local schools from setting stricter rules. For example, some states prohibit the sale of FMNV on campus until 30 minutes after the last lunch period (see Chapter 4 discussion of state and local policies).

The widespread availability of competitive foods and beverages is well documented (Wechsler et al., 2001). They are often sold in the school cafeteria, and they may be offered elsewhere in school buildings, on school grounds, or at school-sponsored events. According to the Government Accountability Office (GAO) report *School Meal Programs* (GAO, 2005), nearly 90 percent of schools offer competitive foods and beverages. Their prevalence means that most students at all age levels have many food choices in the school environment in addition to the federally reimbursable school nutrition programs or the brown bag lunch (Box 3-1).

The array of possibilities was illustrated graphically in a recent GAO report, reproduced here as Figure 3-1.

Table 3-1 shows the percentage of schools where students can purchase specific types of foods and beverages through à la carte sales in the cafeteria or in vending machines, school stores, canteens, or snack bars. For columns 3 and 4 of the table, the original source, Wechsler et al. (2001), reported percentage of schools (data from the Centers for Disease Control and Prevention [CDC]/School Health Policies and Programs Study [SHPPS]) using as a base the number of schools that had a vending machine, school store, canteen, or snack bar. The base of the percentage was converted to represent all schools by multiplying the percentage reported in the original article by the percentage of schools having at least one of these sales venues.

BOX 3-1
Competitive Foods Are Widely Available

National data on the extent to which competitive foods are offered in schools are available from the 2005 Government Accountability Office (GAO) report (and others). The GAO study found that

- 91 percent of high schools, 88 percent of middle schools, and 67 percent of elementary schools offered foods à la carte;
- 91 percent of high schools, 87 percent of middle schools, and 46 percent of elementary schools had food or beverage vending machines that students were allowed to use;
- 54 percent of high schools, 25 percent of middle schools, and 15 percent of elementary schools sold food through a school store or snack bar; and
- Some schools allowed foods to be sold for fund-raising purposes during school meal periods. For example, fund-raising—e.g., seasonal candy sales or bake sales that raise revenues for school organizations—through the sale of foods to students during the school day as allowed in more than 4 out of 10 schools in 2003–2004. These types of fundraisers were permitted in two-thirds of high schools and less than 40 percent of middle and elementary schools.

SOURCE: GAO, 2005.

For example, the source table in the article indicated that 28.8 percent of elementary schools sold 1-percent milk in a vending machine, school store, canteen, or snack bar. However, only 43 percent of elementary schools were reported to have one or more of these sales venues. Therefore, for all schools, the percentage of elementary schools selling 1-percent milk in at least one of these venues is 43 times 0.288, or 12.4 percent, the percentage reported at the top of column 3 of Table 3-1.

The subsequent discussion provides details about competitive food and beverage sales venues and the kinds of foods often available outside the federally reimbursable school nutrition programs. Often, the same types of foods are sold or served to students in different locations, although safety and health factors such as refrigeration and freshness place limitations on distribution. Most high schools offer competitive foods and beverages in one or more of the categories listed in this section. Access to competitive foods and beverages is more limited in elementary schools, but is still very common.

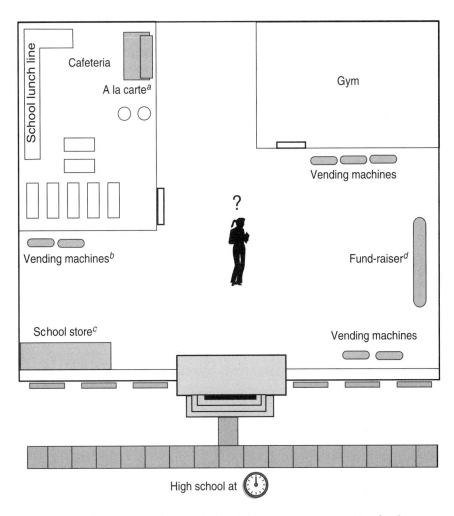

FIGURE 3-1 Groups most frequently involved in various competitive food venues commonly available in high schools.

[a]À la carte: school food authority.

[b]Vending machines: school food authority, vending operator, school official or administrator, physical education department, student association or club.

[c]School store: school official or administrator, student association or club.

[d]Fund-raisers: physical education department, music or art department, business teacher, student association or club, booster groups.

SOURCE: GAO, 2005.

TABLE 3-1 Percentage of Schools Offering Various Types of Competitive Foods by Venue

Type of Food or Beverage	Schools Offering Food or Beverage À La Carte		Schools Where Students Can Purchase Food or Beverage in Vending Machines or in a School Store, Canteen, or Snack Bar	
	Percentage of Elementary Schools	Percentage of Senior High Schools	Percentage of Elementary Schools[a]	Percentage of Senior High Schools[b]
Often Low in Fat				
1% or skim milk	n/a[c]	n/a	12.4	22.7
100% fruit or vegetable juice	57.8	77.4	21.2	63.8
Bottled water	n/a	n/a	13.1	64.7
Bread sticks, rolls, bagels, pita bread, or other bread products	40.9	73.8	6.3	29.1
Fruits or vegetables	68.1	90.4	8.6	21.6
Sandwiches[c]	n/a	n/a	n/a	n/a
Entrées from NSLP meal[c]	n/a	n/a	n/a	n/a
Low-fat cookies, crackers, cakes, pastries, or other low-fat baked goods	36.1	48.0	11.4	48.7
Low-fat or fat-free ice cream, frozen yogurt, or sherbet	27.0	49.0	9.8	24.1
Low-fat or nonfat yogurt	31.0	47.9	5.7	20.5
Salty snacks that are low in fat	29.5	58.3	19.1	63.8
Often High in Fat, Sodium, or Added Sugars				
2% or whole milk	n/a	n/a	21.3	43.7
Chocolate candy	2.4	23.7	12.6	70.9
Cookies, crackers, cakes, pastries, or other baked goods that are not low in fat	48.8	79.9	22.6	79.2
Ice cream or frozen yogurt that is not low in fat	26.3	54.5	13.4	41.7
Other kinds of candy (non-chocolate)	4.2	22.2	15.3	73.7
Salty snacks that are not low in fat	25.8	57.8	21.9	81.5
Soft drinks, sports drinks, or fruit drinks that are not 100% juice	19.0	57.2	25.0	91.9

[a]Among the 43.0 percent of elementary schools with a vending machine, school store, canteen or snack bar.

[b]Among the 98.2 percent of senior high schools with a vending machine, school store, canteen or snack bar.

[c]Not included in survey; data not available.

SOURCE: Derived from Wechsler et al. (2001) with additional information from GAO (2005). Most entries are based on SHPPS (2000) data.

À La Carte Sales

The majority of competitive foods and beverages available during the school day are offered in school cafeterias through à la carte sales. In some cases, à la carte selections are foods and beverages that are also part of a school's regular reimbursable meal offerings. À la carte selections may also include foods and beverages sold separately that are not sold as part of the federally-funded school meals.

As shown in Table 3-1, à la carte sales include a broad range of foods and beverages from fruits, vegetables, and bread products to cookies and salty snacks. It is important to note that the "n/a" symbol in the table means that the relevant food was not asked about in the survey, not that it was not frequently available. Indeed, other information (GAO, 2005) indicates that items not asked about in the survey represented in this table are commonly available à la carte, including milk, bottled water, sandwiches, pizza, and entrées from the main NSLP meals.

Competitive foods, including à la carte offerings, are part of the food service program in a majority of U.S. schools (GAO, 2004). However, some states do not allow à la carte sales as part of the school meal programs, and some limit what can be served. For example, Title 126 of the West Virginia Board of Education Policy 4321.1, requires that only meal components can be sold as à la carte items at breakfast, and only fluid milk, milk shakes, and bottled water can be sold à la carte at lunch (WVDE, 2004).

Vending Machines

Vending machines are common in secondary schools and many elementary schools also allow them on school property (French et al., 2003; Nestle, 2000). CDC (Wechsler et al., 2001) showed that 43 percent of elementary schools, 74 percent of middle schools, and 98 percent of high schools have either a vending machine, a school store, or a snack bar where students can purchase foods and beverages.

The range of food and beverage choices found in vending machines is much narrower than that of the à la carte line (French et al., 2003). This may be due, in part, to the need for refrigeration of fresh food and beverage products. In a GAO report to Congress, the most common types of food and beverage offered in school vending machines were identified as water, fruit and vegetable juices, sports drinks, salty snacks, and soft drinks (GAO, 2005). The most common types of competitive foods offered in high schools through any venue were identified as fruit and vegetable juices, sports drinks, salty snacks, baked goods, sandwiches, pizza, frozen desserts, candy, and soft drinks (GAO, 2005).

In assessing the prevalence of vending machines in schools, it is important to note that, although they are common, there have been attempts to regulate how and when they are used. Some state and local boards of education have created policies that restrict location and times of use. For example, placement of a vending machine near dining areas is sometimes forbidden because machine sales can detract from participation in the federally reimbursable school nutrition programs. Many states and districts have decided to keep all vending machines turned off during regular school hours or until the end of the last lunch period, or prohibit sale of carbonated soft drinks until the end of the school day. Soft drinks are not sold at elementary and middle schools in some states. Many state and district policies that address the content of vending machines specify that foods and beverages sold in them must meet acceptable nutrition guidelines or that at least half of all items in the machines meet nutrition guidelines.

School Stores, Snack Bars, and Related Venues

Other venues for competitive foods and beverages such as school stores, snack bars, and concession stands often raise money for student activities, school-sponsored clubs, and sports teams. School stores and snack bars are often open during lunch periods as well as before and after school.

Concession stands at sports events and other activities outside school hours are popular with booster organizations that rely on the funds garnered from the sale of foods and beverages to support related activities. Relatively few state or district policies address the sale of competitive foods and beverages on school grounds outside the school day. However, wellness policy requirements recently enacted in federal law prompted a number of districts to address food and beverage availability in various venues.

Special Fund-Raisers

In addition to school stores, snack bars, and concession stands, other fund-raising activities may also occur during the school day. These fundraisers may include the sale of foods such as candy bars, cakes, and pizza. They may also include more nutritious foods such as low-fat dairy products, juices, fruits, vegetables, nuts, grain products, meats, and legumes.

Fund-raisers conducted during school hours often follow policies established at the school or state levels for other competitive foods and beverages. Many schools allow food and beverage items to be sold during school lunch periods; others do not allow sales while meals are being served. Some districts have policies that place limitations on the frequency of sales, for example, one event per month during school hours. If a student store operates in the food service area, sales of FMNV are prohibited during meal periods (time of serving and the time that students spend eating meals) by federal regulation.

Foods Used as Rewards and Discipline

Foods and beverages used as rewards for achievement in school are also a form of competitive foods and beverages. For example, a math teacher may include the use of colored candies for props in lessons teaching computation. If the child is successful, he or she may be allowed to eat the candy as a reward. Also, food is used as a reward for good behavior in some classroom situations. Use of food as a reward or for discipline can convey unintended messages about dietary behaviors and may be associated with the development of inappropriate food choices and patterns (Orrell-Valente et al., 2007). Furthermore, use of food as a reward does not model healthful eating behaviors (Ritchie et al., 2005). Some schools have reported that teachers and others use food as an aid in managing behavior and as academic incentives (GAO, 2003). A 2002 survey of 339 Kentucky schools found that "81 percent used food as a reward for behavior, attendance, or academic achievement, and 90 percent used nonfood rewards" (USDA/CDC, 2005).

Although it may be difficult to control the use of food as reward or discipline, some schools have attempted to discourage the use of food as rewards and some district wellness policies have included rules to address this issue.

Effects of Competitive Foods and Beverages on Students' Food Intakes

Substantial proportions of competitive foods and beverages—though not all of them—are of relatively low nutritional quality. This has caused many observers to be concerned that these foods and beverages may have negative effects on the overall quality of students' diets. In the absence of experimental data or large-scale studies, the evidence on this issue must be viewed as suggestive rather than conclusive. The subsequent review includes several selected studies of the nutritional impact of competitive foods and beverages.[1]

Kubik et al. (2003) studied seventh and eighth graders to examine possible displacement of fruits and vegetables by competitive foods and beverages and concluded there was a negative correlation between the number of à la carte items available and the amount of fruits and vegetables children consumed. Also, the presence of snack vending machines on campus was

---

[1]The discussion draws heavily on the similar review in Story et al. (2006, p. 116).

associated with a decline in fruit intake among students compared to those in schools that did not have snack vending machines.

Cullen and Zakeri (2004) found that when children transitioned into middle schools with additional competitive food and beverage options, consumption of fruits, milk, and non-starchy vegetables tended to be lower. Consumption of high-fat vegetables went up.

Templeton et al. (2005) examined sixth graders in three middle schools who sometimes bought competitive foods and beverages, including snack items and sweetened beverages, at school. They found that purchase of these items tended to be associated with higher food energy intakes and higher consumption of fats.

Each of these studies included a relatively small sample, but the results support the view that competitive foods and beverages may be associated with less healthful eating practices at school. It is likely that more studies will become available in the coming years as evaluations are conducted of policies designed to limit the availability of competitive foods and beverages.

Other studies have focused on factors influencing food choice by student age. O'Dea (2003) examined the ability of children and adolescents to select benefits and barriers to healthful food choices and to suggest ways to overcome them. The older students (fifth and sixth grades) were found to be able to articulate the benefits of selecting healthful foods and the adverse effects of non-healthful food choices. Neumark-Sztainer et al. (1999) assessed perceptions about factors influencing food choices among adolescents. This study found a broad range of factors that contributed to food choices, including concern for health. Among the most important factors were food appeal, convenience, and time involved in eating. However, the study also revealed that by addressing the range of factors influencing adolescent food choices, interventions could be designed to improve their choices.

COORDINATING SCHOOL NUTRITION POLICIES WITH OTHER HEALTH-RELATED PROGRAMS IN SCHOOLS

There has been growing awareness among both health professionals and educators that it is important to coordinate school nutrition policies within the broader context of all school health-related programs. In particular, considering these programs in this broader context makes it possible to set priorities and to make sure that the relevant programs work in complementary ways for maximum effectiveness. Described below are components to consider in coordination of health-related policies. More detail is provided about two areas that are particularly closely linked to nutrition policy: physical education and nutrition education.

Growth in Interest in Coordinated School Health Programs

A significant factor contributing to interest in the coordination of school health-related policies is the leadership work of CDC. In particular, since 1994, CDC encouraged schools to use the Coordinated School Health Program (CSHP) model, which consists of eight interactive components: health education; physical education; health services; nutrition services; counseling, psychological, and social services; healthful school environments; health promotion for staff; and family and community involvement. Materials available from CDC encourage schools to further define their comprehensive school health programs.

Increased interest in the coordination of school health-related policies was stimulated by the 2004 reauthorization legislation for the child nutrition programs. This required all school districts that participate in the federal school meal programs to develop local wellness policies by July 1, 2006, setting guidelines for foods and beverages sold and offered in schools, nutrition education, and opportunities for physical activity. Specifically, the law required that local wellness policies include

- Goals for nutrition education, physical activity, and related activities
- Nutrition guidelines for all foods and beverages available at the school during the school day
- An assurance that guidelines for reimbursable meals will not be less restrictive than USDA regulations
- A plan for measuring implementation of the wellness policies
- Involvement of parents, students, and other school constituencies in the wellness policy process

Some school districts completed their wellness policies in 2006, while others are likely to do so soon. This spurred considerable interest and activity among schools in addressing these issues.

It is important to note that the development of wellness policies within schools is relatively recent, and much implementation and monitoring will still be required. This report should be of use to local wellness policy committees and school districts that are still in the process of developing wellness policies, are developing implementation and monitoring procedures for their policies, or are modifying their wellness policies.

Below are overviews of the goals and activities relating to the physical activity and nutrition education elements of these coordinated policies that are particularly germane to the committee's task.

Physical Education

Physical education and related activities are important in a study of competitive foods and beverages because children's physical activity levels are critical to determining their energy expenditures, and thus their food needs. Physical activity is generally accepted as a contributor to good health (IOM, 2002/2005).

National Recommendations Regarding Physical Activity and Education

The DGA (DHHS/USDA, 2005) recommends that children and adolescents engage in at least 60 minutes of physical activity most days of the week. In addition, *Healthy People 2010* (DHHS, 2000) provides two related recommendations:

1. Increase to at least 50 percent the proportion of adolescents who participate in daily physical education.
2. Increase to at least 50 percent the proportion of adolescents who spend at least half their school physical education class time engaged in physically active activities.

The National Association for Sport and Physical Education (NASPE) recommends that all elementary school students participate in at least 150 minutes per week of physical education, and all middle and high school students participate in at least 225 minutes per week for the entire school year (NASPE/AHA, 2006). These recommendations reflect a growing awareness that greater physical activity levels are important both for contributing to children's overall health and reducing the "obesity epidemic."

Current Levels of Physical Activity and Education

Physical education standards and requirements are generally determined at the local level and are based on policies set by individual states or national recommendations. Information compiled by the NASPE (NASPE/ AHA, 2006) indicates that about 70 percent of states mandate physical education for elementary students, while 83 percent of these do so for high school students. However, only about 20 percent specify the number of minutes required, and of the few that do specify time, only two are consistent with the NASPE recommendations.

According to data from the CDC Youth Risk Behavior Survey (Eaton et al., 2006), in 2005, approximately 54 percent of high school students were enrolled in a physical education class, but only about 33 percent of students participated on a daily basis. Only about 84 percent of students were physically active during their physical education classes when participating.

Nutrition Education

Encouraging healthy eating habits at a young age is generally seen as an important contributor to optimal growth, development, health, and well-being and to prevention of some chronic diseases. Schools are in a good position to help young people improve eating habits by implementing effective nutrition education programs and support services (DASH, 2006). Reviews of nutrition education in schools have found that most programs have resulted in moderate to minimal effects, due in some measure to implementation issues and short time frames (Baranowski et al., 2003a, 2003b; Contento et al., 1995; Doak et al., 2006; Flynn et al., 2006; Lytle and Achterberg, 1995; Lytle et al., 2001). However, improved eating patterns are more likely to occur when changes in the school meals are implemented as well as classroom curriculums, as was found, for example, with the Child and Adolescent Trial for Cardiovascular Health (CATCH), a study of third to fifth graders (Luepker et al., 1996), and the Teens Eating for Energy and Nutrition at School (TEENS) study with middle school youth (Lytle et al., 2004). Results of interventions based on changes in the school meals with and without promotional activities (but without a classroom component) found that the use of multiple components was more effective (O'Neil and Nicklas, 2002; Perry et al., 2004; Whitaker et al., 1994). One study found that a curriculum in which students in the classroom cooked the same recipes as offered in the cafeteria resulted in increased consumption of these recipes in the school lunch, whereas changes in the school lunch by itself did not (Liquori et al., 1998). Although nutrition education to enhance healthy eating is challenging even with changes in the school environment (Lytle et al., 2006), this research does suggest that classroom nutrition education can enhance the effectiveness of school-wide efforts to improve children's eating practices.

In light of the above, nutrition education may provide an important opportunity for reinforcement of the importance of, and skills used in, making healthful food choices. Below are highlights of key aspects of nutrition education in the school setting.

National Recommendations Pertaining to Nutrition Education

A position statement issued jointly by the American Dietetic Association, the Society for Nutrition Education, and the American School Food Service Association (now called the School Nutrition Association) calls for comprehensive, sequential nutrition education, spanning preschool through secondary school (Briggs et al., 2003). It also states: "integrating nutrition education topics into other subject instruction areas may be necessary because of the current educational emphasis on academic achievement and mastery of core standards. However, this strategy should complement, not replace, a comprehensive nutrition education program. Multiyear, sequential nutrition curriculums from preschool through grade 12 facilitate the best use of limited instructional time."

In terms of suggested content, the statement recommends nutrition education programs that

- focus on changing specific behaviors rather than learning general facts about nutrition;
- employ active learning or experiential strategies;
- use developmentally appropriate instructional concepts;
- devote adequate time and intensity to focus on behaviors and skills building;
- provide teachers and other staff with adequate training in nutrition education; and
- link with the school environment by involving the child's family and providing school meal programs and school-related policies that reinforce classroom nutrition education.[2]

Current Levels of Nutrition Education in Schools

Few states specifically require nutrition education as a stand-alone curriculum topic. More frequently, the nutrition curriculum is imbedded in general health or science programs and not taught by nutrition specialists (Kann et al., 2001). A CDC survey conducted in 2000, the School Health Policies and Programs Study, found that 69 percent of states required the topic of "nutrition and dietary behavior" to be taught at the elementary, middle, and high school levels. At the elementary, middle, and high school levels, 75 percent, 76 percent, and 82 percent of school districts stated that they required nutrition be taught. The percentages by school for these three levels were 86 percent, 81 percent, and 87 percent, respectively. Education about nutrition and dietary behavior was incorporated into health education courses in middle and high schools about 75 percent of the time, and was incorporated into other courses about 50 percent of the time. The main topics covered were the benefits of healthy eating, the Food Guide Pyramid,

---

[2]Other sets of recommendations in the area include DASH (2006) and National Center for Chronic Disease Prevention and Health Promotion; Healthy Schools, Healthy Youth!; Nutrition Summary.

eating more fruits and vegetables, and balancing food intake and physical activity. These topics were reported to be taught by more than 90 percent of all schools. The major skills taught were decision-making and goal-setting skills for healthy eating (Kann et al., 2001).

The 2004 School Health Profiles survey of public secondary schools in 25 states and 10 large urban school districts found that the percentage requiring any instruction in nutrition and dietary behavior in a mandatory health education course ranged from 93 to 100 percent with a median of about 99 percent (CDC, 2006). However, although some nutrition education appears to be common in schools, the amount offered is often quite limited. The median number of hours per year that schools devote to teaching nutrition and dietary behavior is estimated to be five for elementary schools, four for middle schools, and five for high schools (Kann et al., 2001). Given this very limited time spent on nutrition education, teachers can be encouraged to focus on the importance of a healthy school food environment and skills in making healthy food choices.

A notable trend in nutrition education has been the use of innovative hands-on and behaviorally focused teaching strategies to enhance healthy eating at school. For example, classroom nutrition education curriculums involving cooking have been shown to enhance the consumption of similar foods introduced at the lunch meal (Liquori et al., 1998). Likewise, working in school gardens has been used to promote healthful eating (Graham and Zidenberg-Cherr, 2005). Another program to improve children's diets, increase physical activity, and prevent tobacco use was the CATCH program, implemented in 96 schools in 4 states. Three years after the intervention, the CATCH cohort had maintained the positive outcomes from the program (Hoelscher et al., 2001).

FISCAL CONCERNS

Many school districts feel financial pressure as they strive to achieve the twin goals of having strong academic programs and providing a wide range of extracurricular activities for students. Discussed below are the implications of this issue for policies on competitive foods and beverages.

The past few years have been a time of considerable change in primary and secondary education in the United States, with important implications for school budgets. Most importantly, the No Child Left Behind Act placed pressure on school systems to increase the quality of instruction to ensure that children pass the testing programs mandated by the act. Challenged by these and other instructional pressures, schools have become increasingly creative in funding programs and providing resources that enhance the overall educational environment.

Also important to recognize is that school administrators have limited discretion over how state and federal funds are used. Typically, budget allocations from various funding sources are designated for specific areas such as salaries of instructional staff, textbooks, instructional and library supplies, computers, technology supplies, printing supplies, equipment, furniture, and capital improvements.

Competitive food and beverage revenues may be one of the few sources of discretionary funds for a school administrator. These monies may provide funding for a variety of extracurricular activities such as field trips, art programs, theater, band and orchestra, additional computers and technology equipment, and educational competitions. Although these are items and/or activities that fall outside instructional budget allocations, they can be important in the operation of a successful school.

The revenues generated by sales of competitive foods and beverages are relatively small. Evidence presented below suggests that they probably amount to less than 1 percent of expenditures in most schools. However, as a percentage of the revenues spent on these and similar discretionary activities, the competitive food and beverage revenues may be significant. Below are estimates of the overall size of these revenues.

Revenues Generated by Sales of Competitive Foods and Beverages

The most recent nationally representative source of information of competitive food and beverage finances is a 2005 GAO study. Based on survey reports from a sample of schools in 2003–2004, this report estimated the percentages of schools in various ranges of competitive food and beverage revenues.[3] Assumptions about the average revenues of the schools within each range show the average annual competitive food revenues were $8,500 per school for elementary schools, $39,500 for middle schools, and $80,000 for high schools (see Table 3-2). Extrapolating, based on numbers of schools nationwide, suggests approximately $2.3 billion worth of competitive foods and beverages are sold annually. Several different perspectives can be used to assess this $2.3 billion figure. As a fraction of total school

---

[3]It appears that for à la carte sales, the GAO numbers reflect *gross revenue* from beverage and food sales, but they may reflect something closer to *net revenue* for vending and some other competitive food venues. In defining revenue, the GAO report indicates on p. 27, "Throughout this report, revenue for each type of competitive food venue includes all revenue generated through competitive food sales. We did not ask survey respondents for information on profits retained after covering expenses." However, some ambiguity remains as to what "generated" means. It appears that it means revenue *accruing to the schools*. For à la carte sales, this would be the *total value* of the food and beverage sales, whereas for another major revenue source, vending, the school only receives the payments made to the school by the vendor, which do not include the total value of the food and beverage items sold because they do not include the vendor's costs and profits.

TABLE 3-2 Competitive Foods and Beverages Revenue in Schools

	Elementary	Middle	High	All
Percentage of schools with more than $100,000 revenue from competitive foods and beverages	0%	11%	32%	
Percentage of schools with less than $1,000 revenue from competitive foods and beverages	52%	21%	9%	
Average annual competitive foods and beverages revenue per school[a]	$8,500	$39,500	$80,000	
Approximate number of schools[b]	52,000	16,000	15,000	
Estimated total competitive food revenues across all schools[c]				$2.3 billion
Reference figure: Total expenditures of all schools[d]				$384 billion

[a]Computed assuming that averages were approximated by midpoints of ranges in GAO, 2005, p. 28.
[b]Based on GAO (2005), p. 54.
[c]Extrapolated based on numbers of schools and the average annual competitive foods and beverages revenue per school.
[d]Total expenditures in all U.S. schools for all purposes; based on multiplying an estimate of per pupil annual cost of $8,000, times approximately 48 million pupils.

expenditures, it is quite low—less than 1 percent. However, as a share of the overall money spent on food service in the schools, it is much more substantial. Federal school meal program costs for 2004 are estimated to have been about $9.4 billion (Source: www.fns.usda.gov/pd/cncosts.htm [accessed February 27, 2007]). With the estimated $2.3 billion of competitive foods, this implies a total revenue related to food service of $11.7 billion. Competitive food and beverage sales represents about 19 percent of this figure. To place this number in perspective, the total expenditures on public schools was approximately $384 billion.

A third perspective that may be more meaningful than either of the above is that discussed in GAO (2005). Competitive food monies may be a very important source of revenue for schools because they fund a significant share of discretionary activities that cannot be funded out of regular school activities (see additional discussion below).

In most schools, the majority of competitive food monies is likely to come from à la carte sales in the cafeteria. Data for high schools suggest that à la carte sales make up well over 50 percent of total revenues related to competitive foods and beverages. Similar conclusions can be drawn from the American School Food Service Association's (ASFSA) *À la Carte and Vending Research Program, Summary Report* (ASFSA, 2002). Comparisons between the revenue for à la carte and for vending may be somewhat misleading (see footnote 3).

How the Money Is Used

In assessing how competitive food and beverage funds are used by schools, it is important to distinguish between à la carte sales and revenues and sales from other competitive food and beverage venues. À la carte revenues usually (but not always) accrue to the district SFA, which uses the money to offset deficits in the food service operations or to improve the quality of foods and beverages sold. On the other hand, although revenues from vending and other competitive food and beverage sales venues sometimes accrue to the SFA, they are more likely to accrue to special accounts controlled by school officials for use in supporting various school activities directly to student organizations.[4]

Use of Competitive Foods Money by School Food Service Authority

In the GAO (2003) survey of 22 schools in 13 school districts, SFA indicated that financial pressures have led them to offer more and "less healthful" à la carte items because these items generate needed revenue. "One School Food Service director said that à la carte sales help her balance the budget. She said the SFA probably sells about $600 a day in à la carte items."

Similar information was reported in a 2002 School Nutrition Association (then ASFSA) study on school à la carte and vending sales (ASFSA, 2002). SFA stated that à la carte sales had a number of positive impacts. In particular, study participants reported that the revenue from sales of competitive foods allowed

- more price flexibility and higher pricing margins;
- greater overall revenue;
- opportunities for offering items such as branded foods, which respond to student preferences, but cannot be offered under the standard reimbursable meal; and
- opportunities to be more responsive to student requests in menu offerings.

---

[4]For additional information on the split of monies across different sources, see ASFSA (2002, pp. 27 and 47).

Use of Competitive Foods Money by Other Constituencies in the School

As indicated earlier, schools often find it necessary to identify ways of funding programs and activities that fall outside those areas that receive funding through the instructional supplies and materials budgets.

GAO (2005) (see Figure 3-2) reported that schools use money from the sale of competitive foods and beverages in diverse ways, including funding field trips, school assemblies, athletic facilities and equipment, textbooks, and other supplies. Similar information was reported in the 2005 USDA and CDC *Making It Happen!* toolkit (USDA/CDC, 2005).

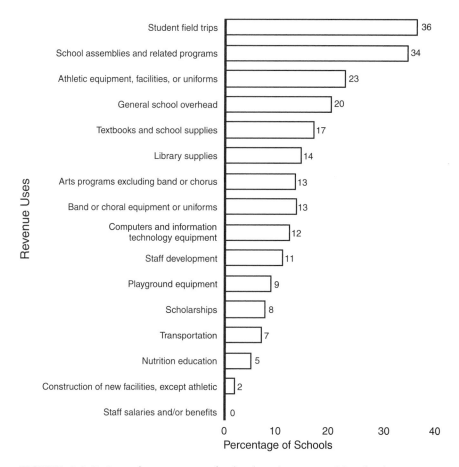

FIGURE 3-2 Estimated percentage of schools using competitive foods revenue, excluding food service revenue, for various purposes in 2003–2004.
SOURCE: GAO, 2005.

Thus à la carte revenues, which are likely the majority of competitive food revenues (see discussion above), are mainly devoted to food service operations. Essentially, they are used to pay off salaries of food service workers and to obtain food and other supplies. As indicated in ASFSA (2002), more than 90 percent of à la carte revenues are used for food service operation costs.

Experience of Schools in Restricting Competitive Foods and Beverages

The committee examined the financial experiences of schools that have restricted the availability of competitive foods and beverages to their students. Relatively little information was available because schools have only recently begun to make this transition and share their experiences (see below).

Evidence from the California LEAF Study

Probably the most thorough research is a pilot study of the effects of competitive food and beverage restriction implementation in California (Woodward-Lopez et al., 2005). Sixteen schools in nine districts were studied, and financial data were obtained from school district personnel. The study was conducted by the Center for Weight and Health at the University of California at Berkeley.

The investigators found that, when competitive food and beverage restrictions were imposed, gross revenue from school meals went up for 13 of 16 schools after the pilot changes. This increase in gross revenue occurred largely because more students participated in the NSLP, instead of buying competitive foods. However, gross revenue by itself is an imperfect measure of impact on the schools because it fails to account for possible changes in costs that might offset the revenue. The investigators found that only 5 of the 16 schools could provide sufficient data with which to estimate changes in *net* income. Net income decreased in two of those five schools and increased in three. For at least one and possibly two of the three schools where net income was increased, other factors, not directly related to restricting competitive foods also seemed to have been at least partially responsible.

Although this study was limited to only 16 schools in a single state, it suggests at least two important conjectures. First, it is unclear that schools can implement changes in competitive foods and beverages without losses in net income. Second, it appears that the routine availability of accounting information in schools is limited, and thus it is difficult to fully assess changes in net income. Research that follows on this pilot study may clarify the impact of changes in competitive food sales on school net income.

2005 GAO Report

GAO (2005) noted concerns about the availability of information to assess the financial impact of competitive food and beverage restrictions. GAO staff visited six schools that had recently undertaken initiatives to improve the quality of competitive foods and beverages, and examined financial impacts. However, they reported, "The effects of changes to competitive foods on revenues were often unclear because of limited data; nonetheless, many officials expressed concern about revenue losses."

Evidence from Trade Sources

The number of school vending machines is reported to have decreased for schools (elementary through college) between 2003 and 2004. Vending operators cited two primary reasons for retreating from schools: (1) resistance from SFA that view vending operations as competition rather than support, and (2) growing nutrition restrictions (Maras, 2004).

School Reports

Additional discussions of the financial effects of implementing new competitive foods policies are also available in *Making It Happen!*, a compendium of 32 school and school district "success stories" published by the government to provide information on how to improve nutrition in the schools. Seventeen of the school district reports mention financial variables, and twelve indicate that limiting competitive foods and beverages did not adversely affect school revenues or resulted in benefit; four reported no change (USDA/CDC, 2005).

School reports are of limited use because the information reflects school and parent self-reports rather than independent outside observations and a standardized research protocol. Also, these school reports were not randomly selected; they were chosen to highlight schools that were changing their competitive foods program. Overall, this compendium suggests that it has been possible to restrict competitive foods and beverages without the school reporting additional financial pressure. However, assessing feasibility across schools will be difficult. Careful consideration must be given to how data are represented. When schools report success or failure, the data reported may not be representative of financial impacts across all schools.

The importance of small revenue sources may be underestimated because school officials often have more discretion over income from competitive foods than over other funding streams. There is insufficient evidence available to determine the financial impact of restricting competitive foods and beverages.

MARKETING

Marketing activities represent another element of the nutrition-related environment in schools. Marketing includes both the selling of specific brands of food and beverages, and the prominent use of food and beverage company names and logos in schools. Although there is a paucity of rigorous scientific evidence on the impact of marketing on food selection and purchase by children in schools, it is possible that marketing reflects, in part, the considerable resources many students have to spend. Food and beverage companies are also eager to shape students' brand awareness and loyalty, and thus purchasing patterns, as they mature into adulthood (GAO, 2000; IOM, 2006; Palmer et al., 2004; Story and French, 2004). For example, more than $200 billion is spent annually by children and adolescents. Candy, carbonated soft drinks, and salty snacks consistently represent the leading categories of food and beverage items that are purchased by this group (IOM, 2006). In addition, a rigorous review of peer-reviewed literature on the effect of food marketing, primarily advertising, found that among many factors, food and beverage marketing influences the preferences and purchase requests of children, influences consumption at least in the short term, is a likely contributor to less healthful diets, and may contribute to negative diet-related health outcomes and risks among children and youth (IOM, 2006). Indeed, in many ways the schools represent an ideal audience for marketing, with millions of students attending school at least six hours a day, five days a week. Schools are often also eager to be involved in marketing efforts to help alleviate chronically tight budgets (Palmer et al., 2004; Story and French, 2004).

The report *Food Marketing to Children and Youth: Threat or Opportunity?* (IOM, 2006) indicates that "[t]he competitive multifaceted marketing of high-calorie and low-nutrient food and beverage products in school settings is widely prevalent and appears to have increased steadily over the past decade." Encouraging soft drink sales is the most common kind of marketing activity in schools. In addition, 20 percent of high schools sell branded fast foods (Wechsler et al., 2001).

A particularly prevalent form of advertising at school is on scoreboards, in the form of corporate logos and soft drink ads (GAO, 2000). Also, more than one-third of middle and high schools use Channel One, which provides news programs for classroom viewing that include commercials for soft drinks and snacks.

Food and beverage marketing in the school environment can appear in many forms. For example, Story and French (2004) identified

- sales of foods and beverages that benefit the school, the school district, or a student activity;

- sales of brand-name fast foods;
- awards to schools of cash or equipment in exchange for proofs of purchase of foods or beverages;
- coupons, labels, or receipts from students;
- fund-raising activities by parents and students that involve the sale of foods and beverages;
- food and beverage advertising in schools, on athletic fields, on buses, and on school equipment and books;
- food and beverage advertising in school publications, on television programs shown at school, and on computers;
- free food and beverage samples;
- educational materials, contests, and grants provided by food and beverage corporations; and
- market research conducted by food and beverage firms at school, concerning student food and beverage preferences.

Many observers have raised concerns about the extent of food and beverage marketing in schools and the susceptibility of students to its influence. Despite this, local, state, or national regulation or voluntary controls on this kind of marketing in schools are not widespread (IOM, 2006). Because the selling of various products in school is itself a form of marketing, the growing restrictions on competitive foods and beverages in schools, as documented in Chapter 4, may be resulting in less marketing overall.

OTHER ASPECTS OF THE SCHOOL ENVIRONMENT RELATED TO THE NSLP AND COMPETITIVE FOODS AND BEVERAGES

Schools vary substantially in many different ways, including physical layout, class and activity scheduling, the availability of various programs, and levels of overall maintenance. Many of these factors have an influence on how the use of competitive foods and beverages has evolved in the schools and on the difficulty of creating standards for such foods and beverages. Noted below are the most important of these interactions.

Lack of Space

Some schools lack the physical capacity to serve all of their students in the available cafeteria space during times generally regarded as appropriate for lunch. As a result, schools have sometimes resorted to beginning the lunch period much earlier than most students might want. This potentially diminishes the attractiveness of participating in the NSLP (and thereby increases the relative appeal of competitive foods and beverages when students are hungry). Other consequences of having inadequate cafeteria space may include overcrowded conditions or the need for students to use other food sources, such as school stores or vending machines, to obtain food, thus increasing the relative attractiveness of competitive foods.

Scheduling

Closely related to issues concerning cafeteria space are broader constraints that schools face for scheduling. Under pressure to ensure high academic performance (or to provide time for other school priorities), some schools schedule relatively short lunch periods. This may lead some students to choose competitive foods and beverages rather than NSLP meals if these can be purchased more quickly. A related timing issue involves whether schedules are such that students choose between buying and consuming an NSLP meal or having more recess time. Also, for high school students, there may be choices between having time for lunch and having time for an extra class or other academic opportunity.

Open Versus Closed Campuses

Some schools, particularly high schools, choose to "open" their campuses to allow students to be away from school during lunch periods and, in some instances, during other times when the students do not have classes scheduled. Nationally, 94 percent of elementary, 89 percent of middle, and 73 percent of high schools have closed campuses (Wechsler et al., 2001). Some schools have an open campus because of space constraints such as those noted above; in other instances, the school district may have made a conscious decision to allow older students to come and go from campus based on the assumption that they have a higher level of responsibility.

The open campus environment affects the dynamic of the interaction between the NSLP and competitive foods and beverages. In large part this is true because being able to leave the campus at lunchtime opens up additional lunch alternatives, thus reducing student use of both the NSLP and school competitive foods and beverages. Having an open campus likely undermines the nutrition objectives of the NSLP, because the foods and beverages bought by students off campus are probably not as nutritious as those served within the NSLP.

Availability of "Grab and Go" Programs Within the NSLP

To compensate for facility constraints and other issues, some schools have developed "express" versions of the NSLP that provide students with meals more quickly. Similar efforts to serve meals more quickly include "grab and go" breakfasts and breakfasts in the classroom. These alternatives allow students the opportunity to select options that are more nutritious and decrease opportunities to select competitive foods and beverages of low nutritional value.

Conditions Within the School Cafeteria

Students use of competitive foods and beverages may also be influenced by school cafeteria conditions. Besides overcrowding, key issues include cleanliness, noise levels, and the enforcement of rules that ensure a pleasant, safe eating environment without being overly restrictive. A related issue is the availability of alternative places to eat within the school or on the school grounds, and whether students are allowed to consume NSLP meals and/or foods and beverages at non-cafeteria locations.

In summary:

1. Most schools have the infrastructure or arrangements in place to produce and serve healthy foods, either through their own kitchens, central district kitchens, or outside vendors. Although compliance is not yet 100 percent, evidence shows that greater numbers of schools are meeting the nutritional standards for the NSLP and SBP in meals served.

2. The successful operation of the NSLP and SBP in most schools, with their extensive nutritional requirements, suggests that schools have the capability to shift from current competitive foods and beverages to more nutritious competitive foods and beverages.

3. At a time when there are significant pressures on SFA budgets, competitive foods and beverages may be important for many SFAs to meet requirements that they balance their budgets. This may be an obstacle to modifying school competitive food and beverage policies in some schools.

SUMMARY

The preceding discussion of ways in which the school environment influences competitive food and beverage use is not exhaustive. However, it highlights the most important interactions, including the fact that different school conditions lead to quite different patterns of competitive food and beverage use. It also suggests that the effects of regulating competitive foods and beverages may also "play out" differently depending on the circumstances.

4

Foods and Beverages Sold Outside the School Meal Program: Federal, State, Local, and Industry Initiatives

INTRODUCTION

The school food environment has a large impact on the dietary intake of children and adolescents because a substantial proportion of total daily energy is consumed at school. National data show that foods eaten at school comprise 19 to 50 percent of students' total daily energy intake (Gleason and Suitor, 2001). Foods and beverages at school are available through the U.S. Department of Agriculture (USDA) federally reimbursable school nutrition programs, that is, school breakfast and lunch programs, and also through competitive foods and beverages from à la carte lines in cafeterias, vending machines, snack bars, and other venues. Although school breakfasts, school lunches, and federally funded after-school snack and meal programs must meet federal nutrition standards to receive federal subsidies, competitive foods and beverages are largely exempt from such requirements. However, state and local authorities can impose additional restrictions. In response to growing concerns about childhood obesity, there has been national attention for the need to establish school nutrition standards and to restrict access to high-calorie, nutrient-poor competitive foods and beverages. As a result, over the past few years, school nutrition policy initiatives are in place at the federal, state, and local levels and there have been positive industry responses. The following is a background on the history of federal legislation and regulation of competitive foods and beverages and examination of recent federal, state, local, and industry policy initiatives related to competitive foods and beverages in schools.

History of Federal Legislation and Regulation of Competitive Foods

Competitive foods have been a controversial issue for more than 35 years. The Child Nutrition Act of 1966 (Pub. L. No. 89–642) authorized the Secretary of Agriculture to promulgate regulations necessary to carry out the mission of the government for child nutrition programs. In 1970, out of concern for the growing trend of "junk foods" (foods of minimal nutritional value) being offered in the public schools, the Child Nutrition Act (Pub. L. No. 91–248) was amended to give the Secretary authority to issue a regulation concerning competitive foods (Griffith et al., 2000). The resulting regulation stipulated that (1) competitive foods and beverages available in cafeterias during meal periods had to contribute to reimbursable meals; (2) the revenue from competitive food sales would accrue to the nonprofit food service account; and (3) food and beverage sales elsewhere in the school could not occur at times and places that competed with the federally reimbursable lunch program (Garnett et al., 2006). As a result of this amendment, many schools lost revenues on which they had come to depend. In 1972, in response to pressure from the school community, student organizations, and companies selling foods and beverages to schools, Congress once again amended the Child Nutrition Act (Pub. L. No. 92–433) to permit revenue from competitive foods and beverages to accrue to the school, approved school organizations, or the school's food service unit (Griffith et al., 2000). This change resulted in an increased presence of vending machines and other competitive food and beverage venues in schools to gain revenue for school activities. The 1973 regulation also directed state agencies to establish regulations and instructions to control the sale of competitive foods and beverages.

In 1977, due to concerns about the quality of children's diets and inconsistent state regulations, Congress amended Pub. L. No. 95–166 to stipulate that the sale of competitive foods and beverages was subject to approval by the U.S. Secretary of Agriculture (Garnett et al., 2006; Griffith et al., 2000). This statute gave the secretary authority to regulate which items would be allowed as competitive foods. In April 1978, USDA proposed a rule that established a definition for nutritious and non-nutritious foods. This proposed rule prohibited the sale of foods in four categories: all candy, soda water (soft drinks), frozen desserts, and chewing gum. However, there were no nutrition standards for these categories. Sales of these items were prohibited throughout the school until after the last lunch period (GAO, 2004). In response to this proposed rule, USDA received more than 2,100 comments, of which 80 percent were in favor of the proposed rule. Of these, 40 percent wanted the list of prohibited foods expanded or the time restrictions on sales extended (Garnett et al., 2006). In December 1978, USDA withdrew the rule to consider strengthening it and to provide additional opportunity for public participation in the rule-making process. USDA then held a series of public hearings responding to a series of questions disseminated through the *Federal Register*. In response, USDA received 4,200 comments; of these, roughly 40 percent recommended additional restrictions (Garnett et al., 2006). The final rule in January 1980 restricted the sale of foods of minimal nutritional value (FMNV) in the same four categories (candy, soda water, frozen desserts, and chewing gum) as the 1978 proposal. The final rule also provided specific nutrition criteria for FMNV, which were defined as providing less than 5 percent of the U.S. Recommended Dietary Allowance (RDA) per serving for seven key nutrients (protein, vitamin A, vitamin C, niacin, riboflavin, thiamin, and calcium). The final rule also prohibited the sale of FMNV from the beginning of the school day until after the last lunch period throughout the school (GAO, 2004).

In January 1980, the Community and Nutrition Institute challenged the final regulations as not being restrictive enough. In May 1980, the National Soft Drink Association (NSDA) filed suit in the U.S. District Court against the Secretary of Agriculture on the grounds that the Secretary had exceeded the powers given to him by Congress (Griffith et al., 2000). NSDA challenged the regulations as "arbitrary, capricious, an abuse of discretion, and otherwise not in accordance with law," and requested the court issue a preliminary injunction on implementation of the rule. In June 1980, the U.S. District Court consolidated both cases, denied the request for a preliminary injunction, and dismissed both actions. NSDA appealed the decision to the District of Columbia Court of Appeals (Garnett et al., 2006).

School districts also challenged the proposed rule. In August 1980, the Pulaski County School District in Little Rock, Arkansas "challenged the rule by offering free carbonated beverages, which students could choose instead of milk. USDA attempted to restrict the practice and the Pulaski County School District filed suit against USDA. The court ruled in the district's favor" (Garnett et al., 2006).

In 1983, NSDA won their appeal based on what has become known as the "time and place" rule. The Court of Appeals ruled that the congressional intent was to prohibit the restricted foods only in the food service areas during meal periods. In 1984, USDA proposed to revise the regulations to prohibit the sale of FMNV within food service areas during meal periods. The final rule in 1985: established four categories of FMNV (soft drinks, water ices, chewing gum, and certain candies); specified nutrition criteria as providing less than 5 percent of the U.S. RDA for the key nutrients identified above; prohibited the sale of FMNV within the food service areas during meal periods; and specified that states and local districts may impose additional restrictions (Garnett et al., 2006). The 1985 ruling remains in effect today.

CONCERNS ABOUT COMPETITIVE FOODS

As discussed in Chapter 2, competitive foods are widely available to students in multiple school venues. They have increased in availability in the past five years. Many of these foods and beverages are low in nutritional value and high in sugar, fat, and calories, with the most common being soft drinks, fruit drinks that are not 100 percent juice, salty snacks, high-fat baked goods, and french fries (GAO, 2004; Wechsler et al., 2001).

Several concerns have been raised about competitive foods. Federally reimbursable school meals in the National School Lunch Program (NSLP) and School Breakfast Program (SBP) are required to meet federal nutrition guidelines and comply with the Dietary Guidelines for Americans (DGA) (DHHS/USDA, 2005). School lunches must provide one-third of the RDA for protein, energy, and key vitamins and minerals, and school breakfasts must provide one-fourth of the same nutrients. School meals must also meet the DGA for fat and saturated fat (see Chapter 2). However, these nutrition standards do not apply to à la carte foods and beverages available in the school cafeteria, nor do they apply to other foods and beverages sold throughout the school in vending machines, school stores, snack bars, or fund-raising activities.

The definition of FMNV is narrow and restricts only a small range of competitive foods from being sold during meal times in food service areas. The definition of prohibited foods has not been updated in more than 20 years, and omits many high-calorie foods low in nutrients. Organizations and advocacy groups have called on Congress and USDA to update nutrition standards for foods and beverages available outside the federally reimbursable school nutrition programs (APHA, 2003; NANA, 2005; Trust for America's Health, 2006). A further concern is that, although the federal school meal programs set appropriate portion sizes, competitive foods are offered without serving size guidelines (e.g., students have access to large portions of soft drinks, cookies, french fries, or chips).

A major concern among school food authorities is that the wide availability and promotion of competitive foods in schools diminishes the ability of school meals to deliver on the nation's commitment to provide nutritious meals to children (Griffith et al., 2000; USDA, 2001). The amount of federal money contributed to the NSLP and SBP was $8.8 billion in the 2004–2005 school year and represents a significant investment in children's nutritional health (FRAC, 2006).

School meals can make an important contribution to the nutrition intake of school-age children. Gleason and Suitor (2001) examined intake data from the 1994–1996 Continuing Survey of Food Intakes by Individuals (CSFII) for associations between participation in federally reimbursable school meal programs and dietary intake among school-age children. This study found that children who ate school lunches and breakfasts had higher intakes of nutrients, both at mealtime and as total daily intake, compared to those who did not eat school meals. The study also concluded that their findings were suggestive that participation in the school meal programs declined with increasing availability of competing food options such as à la carte service, vending machines, and school stores. Neumark-Sztainer et al. (2005) studied associations between consumption patterns among high school students and vending machine purchases, and how school policies affect the school food environment. This study found that school policies limiting the hours of operation of snack and soft drink vending machines were associated with a decline in purchases, thus limiting access to foods and beverages high in fat and sugar.

In a Report to Congress (USDA, 2001), USDA highlighted four major concerns about competitive foods:

1. Diet-related health risks. Many competitive foods and beverages are low in nutrient density and high in fat, sugar, and calories, and can negatively affect children's diets and increase risk of excess weight gain.

2. Stigmatization of school meal programs. Low-income children can receive free or reduced-priced school meals. However, only children with money can purchase competitive foods and beverages. Therefore, children may perceive that school meals are primarily for poor children rather than nutrition programs for all children.

3. Impact on school meal programs. The increase in the sale of competitive foods and beverages is associated with a decrease in student participation in the reimbursable school meal program, which may affect the viability of the program. Although à la carte sales bring additional revenues to school food service programs, declining participation results in decreased cash and commodity support. States with more restrictive competitive food and beverage policies have rates of school meal participation that are higher than the national average.

4. Mixed messages. When children are taught in the classroom about good nutrition and healthy food choices, but are surrounded by vending machines, school stores, and à la carte service offering primarily foods of low nutritional value, this sends an inconsistent message about the importance of nutrition.

FEDERAL INITIATIVES

The widespread and unrestricted availability of competitive foods has led many nutrition and health organizations and advocacy groups to recommend setting nutrition standards for foods and beverages offered in schools, and establishing tighter controls of competitive foods and beverages. USDA has urged Congress to take action to foster a healthier school environment by strengthening the statutory language to ensure that (1) all foods and beverages sold or served anywhere in school during the school day meet nutrition standards, and (2) revenue from all competitive food and beverage sales throughout the school accrue to the school food service account (USDA, 2001).

In March 2007, the Child Nutrition Promotion and School Lunch Protection Act of 2007 was introduced in both houses of Congress to amend the Child Nutrition Act of 1966 to improve the nutrition and health of school-age children by having USDA update the definition of FMNV and applying those standards everywhere on school grounds, including in vending machines, à la carte or snack lines, snack bars, and school stores. School-sponsored fund-raisers are exempt in this bill.

A recent federal policy initiative that has implications for competitive foods and beverages in schools emerged from the WIC (Child Nutrition and Women, Infants, and Children) Reauthorization Act of 2004. This Act contains a local school wellness policy provision, a new tool to address obesity and promote healthy eating and physical activity in the school environment. The wellness policy provision required every school district in the country that participates in the federal school meal program to enact a wellness policy by the first day of the 2006–2007 school year. The school district policies must address goals for nutrition guidelines for all foods available at school, nutrition education and physical activity goals, assurances that school meal guidelines are not less restrictive than federal requirements, and plans for evaluating implementation of the policy. The development of the local school wellness policy had to involve parents, students, school food service, and school administrators.

Because the school wellness policies only recently went into effect, little is known at this time about implementation, compliance, or their impact. A preliminary analysis of local wellness policies collected from 112 school districts in 42 states found that only half of the newly approved policies met all of the minimum guidelines for nutrition and physical activity (Source: www.actionforhealthykids.org [Accessed October 10, 2006]). Compliance with the federal policy guidelines varied among school districts. Forty percent did not specify who was responsible for implementation, 19 percent did not address implementation or evaluation, and 14 percent did not specify goals for nutrition education. The School Nutrition Association assessed key characteristics of local wellness policies approved by the school districts with the 100 highest enrollments in the U.S. They found that 99 percent of the schools addressed school meal nutrition standards, and 92–93 percent addressed nutrition standards for foods and beverages in à la carte services and vending machines. The School Nutrition Association has made plans to evaluate the implementation phase of local wellness policies.

STATE AND LOCAL SCHOOL INITIATIVES

According to federal regulations, states and local districts may impose further restrictions on all foods and beverages on school grounds. In response to growing concerns over childhood obesity, there have been widespread efforts to regulate competitive foods and beverages at the state and local levels. Many states, local school districts, and individual schools have implemented competitive food policies that are more restrictive than USDA regulations, though they differ in the type and extent of restrictions. State and local policy initiatives related to competitive foods include the areas of establishing nutritional standards for foods and beverages in schools, restricting access to and sales of competitive foods and beverages, and banning or limiting access to items in vending machines (HPTS, 2005a).

State-Level Policies

Detailed state-level analyses conducted by the Health Policy Tracking Service[1] (HPTS) show that, as of February 2007, approximately half (27) of all states have adopted competitive school food and beverage policies, federal regulations through legislative bills, executive orders, rules, and regulations that are more restrictive than USDA. These include policies that limit the times or types of competitive foods available for sale in vending machines, cafeterias, school stores, and snack bars. Of these, 16 states currently require nutritional standards for competitive foods and beverages at school (Alabama, Arizona, California, Connecticut, Hawaii, Illinois, Kentucky, Louisiana, Maine, New Jersey, New Mexico, North Carolina, Rhode Island, Tennessee, Texas, and West Virginia) (HPTS, 2007). Access to competitive foods is also prohibited by 25 states at certain times during the day or the entire school day, although the time restrictions, type of food/beverage prohibited, and grade level included vary widely. Portion size restrictions of competitive foods or beverages are specified in 14 states (Alabama, Alaska, Arkansas, California, Connecticut, Illinois, Kentucky, Louisiana, New Jersey, North Carolina, Rhode Island, Tennessee, Texas, and West Virginia) (HPTS, 2007). For a state-by-state profile, see Table C-1 in Appendix C.

Over the past few years, state legislative activity in the area of school nutrition has been brisk. In 2004, HPTS noticed a considerable increase in the amount of legislation introduced related to improving the school food

---

[1]The Health Policy Tracking Service (Thomson West, Inc.) identifies, analyzes, and reports on state and federal legislation and policies affecting health services. HPTS also conducts custom policy research and analysis projects, such as state legislation and policies affecting nutrition and physical activity of children and adolescents supported by the Robert Wood Johnson Foundation.

environment, and this issue continues to receive attention in statehouses around the country (HPTS, 2005a). In 2004, 37 states introduced legislation that provided some level of nutritional guidance or encouraged schools to set standards, and measures were enacted in 12 states (HPTS, 2004). In comparison, in 2005, 42 states introduced approximately 200 bills related to nutrition standards, and measures were enacted in 21 states (HPTS, 2005b). In 2006, 31 states introduced or carried over school nutrition legislation and 11 states adopted legislation (HPTS, 2007). Of the 31 states, at least 23 introduced or carried over legislation that would establish or amend school nutrition standards (HPTS, 2007).

The Center for Science in the Public Interest (CSPI) issued a report in 2006 evaluating the policies for foods and beverages sold outside the NSLP for 50 states and the District of Columbia (CSPI, 2006). State policies were graded based on five areas: beverage nutrition standards; food nutrition standards; grade level(s) to which policies apply; time during the school day to which policies apply; and location(s) on campus to which policies apply. The report concluded that although changes are occurring at the state level, such changes are "fragmented, incremental, and not happening quickly enough to reach all schools in a timely way. The nation has a patchwork of policies addressing the nutritional quality of school foods and beverages and the majority of states have weak policies" (CSPI, 2006).

Lawmakers and citizens tend to be divided on the role that states should have in setting nutrition requirements for elementary, middle, and high school students. Some argue that policies should be made at the local level with school administrators, school boards, and parents. Others maintain that state governments, which incur a significant proportion of rising health care costs, should facilitate healthy school nutrition environments (HPTS, 2006). Financial pressures are reported to be the major obstacles to passing legislative mandates (HPTS, 2006). Competitive food sales generate revenue streams for schools, and school and state officials often express concern about legislative measures that would reduce additional sources of income (HPTS, 2006). However, as is evident from the flurry of activity, states continue to press forward.

State policies for competitive foods tend to be most restrictive for elementary schools and least restrictive for high schools. High schools have many more vending machines and competitive food sales, thus more profits and revenues than elementary and middle schools. For example, the 2000 federal School Health Policies and Programs Study (SHPPS) found that 43 percent of elementary schools, 74 percent of middle schools, and 98 percent of high schools have vending machines, school snack bars, or other food sources outside the federally reimbursable school nutrition programs (Wechsler et al., 2001). A recent survey of 40 California secondary schools found that high schools provided students with the greatest access to competitive foods. The survey also found that "nine times more high schools than middle schools had food vending machines, and three times more high schools had a school store compared to middle schools" (Samuels and Associates, 2006). In spite of greater access to competitive foods in middle and high schools, there has been a tendency for nutrition standards for competitive foods to be most restrictive in elementary schools and less so in middle and high schools.

State departments of education have also been involved in initiatives to create healthy school environments. A number of measures have directed state departments of education or, in fewer cases, the U.S. Department of Agriculture to develop rules or recommendations for schools to follow. In 2004, the Texas Department of Agriculture issued a public school nutrition policy for all schools participating in the federal school meal programs (HPTS, 2004). The policy restricted the availability of FMNV and set nutritional standards, as well as portion size restrictions. In addition, the policy limited availability of soft drinks in high schools to 30 percent of all beverages offered, and restricted access to such beverages in middle schools until the end of the last lunch period (HPTS, 2004). In 2005, seven states (Arizona, Kansas, Kentucky, Maine, New Mexico, North Carolina, and South Carolina) mandated that their departments of education develop minimum standards for all foods and beverages sold or served in elementary, middle, or high schools. Kentucky is unique in that in its state school nutrition bills, penalties were established for schools that were not compliant with the new standards. Many of the state initiatives on competitive foods have been in place only for short periods of time, so their impact is unknown. The extent to which these changes may affect rates of childhood obesity, children's diets, or academic performance has not been evaluated. Few systems are in place to evaluate the implementation or effectiveness of these programs. State policies vary widely in scope and requirements, thus representing a mix of policies implemented in isolation. It is therefore hard to get an overall picture of the similarities and differences among states and determine which initiatives are having the most positive effect. Furthermore, with so many different state nutrition standards, specifying differing amounts of fats, sugars, and portion sizes, it may be difficult for food companies to package and formulate products.

Local-Level Policies

In addition to action at the state level, several school districts have joined the growing movement to restrict competitive foods and beverages in schools. More than half of the 10 largest U.S. school districts have policies that go beyond federal and state regulations in restricting competitive foods in schools. For example, starting in the fall of 2003, the New York City Public School District, the largest school district in the country, eliminated candy, soft drinks, and other snack foods from vending machines on school grounds. Vending machines are now limited to selling water, low-fat snacks, and 100 percent fruit juices (GAO, 2004). The Los Angeles Unified School District, the second-largest school district in the country, passed a ban on vending of soft drinks that went into effect in January 2004. In addition, a ban on fried chips, candy, and other snack foods in school vending machines and school stores went into effect July 2004 (GAO, 2004). In 2004, The Chicago Public Schools, the nation's third largest school district, announced a plan to ban soft drinks, candy, and high-fat snacks from school vending machines and replace them with healthier offerings (Story et al., 2006). The Philadelphia School District has a comprehensive school nutrition policy that includes nutrition education components, guidelines for all foods and beverages sold in schools, family and community involvement, and program evaluation (Story et al., 2006).

In 2004 Greves and Rivara (2006) interviewed representatives of school districts with the largest student enrollment in each state and the District of Columbia about nutrition policies concerning competitive foods. The 51 districts accounted for 5.9 million students, representing 11 percent of U.S. students. Of the 51 districts, 39 percent exceeded state or federal requirements in their competitive food policies. Standards specific to grade level were set by 53 percent. Most districts reported having content criteria for competitive food and beverages and prohibited soft drinks. Approximately half of all district policies had restrictions on portion size of foods or beverages. These applied more often to vending machines, à la carte sales, and student stores than to fund-raising activities. Less than a third of policies addressed either monitoring or consequences for failing to monitor.

Another recent survey also looked at competitive food policies in U.S. schools. At the request of Congress, the Government Accountability Office (GAO) conducted a study in 2004–2005 using a random stratified sample of U.S. schools (GAO, 2005). Among the 317 school principals in the survey, 60 percent reported that they had policies in place restricting student access to competitive foods and beverages. The policies were most often developed and enacted at the school district level. Neumark-Sztainer et al. (2005) examined high school students' lunch patterns and vending machine purchases in association with school food policies. In schools with established policies, students reported consuming fewer competitive foods than students in schools without policies. These findings provide evidence that school food policies that decrease access to less nutritious competitive foods are associated with less frequent consumption of these foods during the school day.

Barriers and Lessons Learned

Barriers that have been examined in adopting and implementing school competitive food policies include the major obstacle cited among school nutrition representatives for school districts: the financial impact of limiting competitive foods, specifically soft drinks (Greves and Rivara, 2006). Little reliable data are available on how changes to competitive food sales affect revenues. Detailed revenue records are often not available, but limited data suggest that districts experience mixed revenue effects (GAO, 2005; USDA/CDC, 2005).

Other barriers include a lack of priority among school district administrators to address child nutrition compared to academic achievement benchmarks, and parents and students who resist changes in food choices (Greves and Rivara, 2006). The GAO report found that many people, including district and local officials as well as members of groups selling food in schools, have decision-making responsibility for competitive food and beverage sales and what to sell; but commonly, no one person had responsibility over all sales in a school, making implementation and policy decisions difficult (GAO, 2005). The new federally mandated school wellness policies should facilitate efforts in this area. Another barrier faced by local school districts in making school food policies is that they typically do not determine nutrition criteria and they lack recommended nutrition standards for competitive foods (GAO, 2005).

Many schools throughout the country have made changes to improve the school food environment. *Making It Happen! School Nutrition Success Stories*, a joint project of the Centers for Disease Control and Prevention (CDC) and the USDA Team Nutrition (USDA/CDC, 2005), tells the stories of 32 schools and school districts that have implemented innovative strategies to improve the nutritional quality of foods and beverages sold in schools outside of the federally reimbursable meal programs. The document describes six key approaches for improving the nutritional quality of competitive foods: establish nutrition standards for competitive foods; influence food and beverage contracts; make more healthful foods and beverages available; adopt marketing techniques to promote healthful choices; limit student access to competitive foods; and use fund-raising activities and rewards that support student health. A major finding from *Making It Happen!* is that students will buy and consume healthy foods and beverages and that schools can make money from selling healthful options.

Making It Happen! provides key lessons learned, including the following (1) a single "champion," such as a parent, food service manager, or school principal, is usually the driving force behind the change; (2) because improving school nutrition involves multiple steps, teams with diverse skills and backgrounds are well positioned to undertake such change; (3) a useful starting point is to assess the current nutrition environment of the school to identify strengths and weaknesses; (4) data are needed to document impact and change; and (5) change is a destination and a process. Adopting a nutrition policy does not guarantee it will be implemented; it will require ongoing attention.

NONGOVERNMENTAL AND INDUSTRY INITIATIVES

The Alliance for a Healthier Generation is a nongovernmental program jointly founded by the William J. Clinton Foundation and the American Heart Association and sponsored by the Robert Wood Johnson Foundation to help schools provide a healthful environment for school-age children by assisting schools in setting and meeting standards for improving the health of children in schools. Focus areas include

1. goals to improve the nutritional value of foods served;
2. goals to increase physical activity during the school day and after school;
3. goals for implementation of classroom lessons on healthy lifestyles; and
4. programs for staff wellness.

The Alliance's Guidelines for Competitive Foods for K–12 Schools, released in 2006, are shown in Appendix D.

Industry Initiatives

The food and beverage industries historically have opposed federal or state school nutrition legislation that restricts access to certain foods and beverages, emphasizing that a healthy diet can include all foods and beverages in moderation (HPTS, 2006). However, in the past year, the beverage industry has recognized that it has a role in preventing childhood obesity (HPTS, 2005b). The food and beverage industry has the opportunity to reformulate products and develop new ones to comply with standards.

Steps Toward Improving the Nutritional Value of Foods

In August 2005, in response to growing pressure from parents and public health advocates, the American Beverage Association (ABA) announced a new voluntary school vending policy. ABA asked the beverage industry and school districts to implement the following guidelines: (1) provide only water and 100-percent juice to elementary schools; (2) provide only nutritious and/or lower calorie beverages such as water, 100-percent juice, sports drinks, nonnutritive sweetened soft drinks, and low-calorie juice drinks; sugar-sweetened soft drinks and juice drinks containing 5 percent or less juice would be provided only after school to middle schools; (3) provide a variety of beverage choices, with no more than 50 percent of the vending selections being soft drinks to high schools (ABA, 2005). The policy applied to new contracts, not existing ones.

In May 2006, new school beverage guidelines were announced by the country's top three soft drink companies, Coca-Cola, PepsiCo, Inc., and Cadbury Schweppes, which together control more than 90 percent of school beverage sales. These three companies and ABA established new voluntary guidelines to limit portion sizes and reduce the number of calories available to children during the school day (ABA, 2006). The agreement, assisted by the Alliance for a Healthier Generation, stated that students in elementary schools would be served only bottled water; low-fat and nonfat milk with up to 150 calories per 8 ounces; and 100-percent fruit juice up to 8 ounces. High schools would be allowed to sell bottled water; no or low-calorie beverages with up to 10 calories per 8 ounces; nonfat and low-fat regular and flavored milk with up to 150 calories per 8 ounces; 100-percent juice with no added sweeteners with up to 120 calories per 8 ounces; and light juice and sports drinks with no more than 66 calories per 8 ounces. At least 50 percent of beverages must be water and a no or low-calorie option. Fully implementing the agreement is anticipated to take 3 years, with 75 percent of schools participating by fall 2008 and all by 2009. The guidelines are voluntary, and the success of the program depends on the schools' willingness to amend existing contracts (Burros and Warner, 2006). A progress report on the agreement will be provided at the end of each school year, beginning in 2007 (Burros and Warner, 2006).

In October 2006, the Alliance for a Healthier Generation announced a collaboration with five of the nation's leading food manufacturers to establish voluntary guidelines for foods offered for sale in schools outside of the NSLP to students before, during, and after the school day. Kraft Foods Inc., Mars Inc., Campbell Soup Co., Dannon, and PepsiCo Inc., agreed to begin promoting snacks that meet nutrition guidelines backed by the American Heart Association. The guidelines provide nutrition criteria for total, saturated, and trans fats; sugar; and sodium. Because the guidelines are voluntary, the plan's success will depend on participation of schools in implementing the guidelines (Alliance for a Healthier Generation, 2006). Appendix D shows the food and beverage criteria proposed by the Alliance for a Healthier Generation.

5

Recommended Standards and Actions for Competitive Foods in Schools

INTRODUCTION

This chapter presents the committee's recommended nutrition standards for competitive foods and beverages in schools. As will be discussed in detail below, the committee's recommendations depend on the interactions of a number of important factors that describe competitive foods, including

- types of foods;
- nutrient content of foods and beverages;
- type of schools to which a given standard applies (elementary, middle, or high);
- time of day that a standard applies (school day, after school); and
- competitive food and beverage venues in the school (including use of à la carte versus other sales locations).

To make it possible to develop recommendations in the context of this complexity, it is important to set up a clear framework for presenting detailed recommendations. First, two key underlying working principles on which the committee's recommendations are premised are presented below. Next, a brief overview of the overall approach to the standards is discussed. This overview provides a useful context within which subsequent, more detailed material is presented and interpreted. Finally, a set of working definitions that are important in defining standards are developed, followed by the recommended standards.

Two Key Premises

To understand the committee's proposed nutrition standards for competitive foods, it is useful to highlight 2 of the 10 Guiding Principles defined in Chapter 1 because they particularly direct the committee's recommendations. These key premises, within the context of the Guiding Principles as a whole, are the necessity of using standards based on individual foods rather than the whole diet (Guiding Principle 8), and identification of the *Dietary Guidelines for Americans* (DGA) as the primary source informing the committee's recommendations on specific food components (Guiding Principle 9).

The Necessity of Using Food-Based Standards

As noted in Guiding Principle 8, nutrient standards for competitive foods and beverages must be *food* based, rather than based on overall dietary intake (diet based). This is in contrast to the context of other nutrition policies (e.g., the DGA), in which diet-based standards are the approach of choice. When feasible, a diet-based standard is preferred because this approach recognizes that an individual's health is influenced by the overall pattern of foods consumed, rather than just on individual foods and beverages.

However, unlike the federally reimbursable school nutrition programs, which have some flexibility in meeting intake requirements over time, competitive foods are usually offered and purchased individually without taking into account other daily intake. In this context, each food and beverage must be regarded separately; thus the committee's recommendations set standards for the *individual* foods and beverages. Furthermore, the standards assure that each snack, food, and beverage item offered separately from the federally reimbursable school nutrition programs is consistent with the dietary pattern and specific nutrient recommendations of the DGA, and the committee's rationale for its application of the DGA is explained in the relevant sections of the text. The recommended nutrition standards are based on the assumption that meals are the primary nutrient and calorie source for children for the day. Competitive foods are offered as discretionary calories.

Reliance on the 2005 Dietary Guidelines

As noted in Guiding Principle 9, the majority of recommendations are derived from the summary volume of the DGA (DHHS/USDA, 2005). The committee identified the DGA as the primary resource for formulating its recommendations because they provide the most current guidance for achieving a healthful diet for Americans over the age of 2 years.

Although the scope of the DGA is quite broad, it does not cover all areas of importance to the committee's work on nutrition standards for schools—for example, it lacks recommendations concerning caffeine and nonnutritive sweeteners. Accordingly, the committee supplemented information from the DGA with reviews of original literature and other relevant sources, including the U.S. Government Accountability Office Reports to Congress (GAO, 2003, 2004, 2005). The committee also sought compelling refutation of specific DGA guideline recommendations for school-age children; no such evidence was found.

OVERVIEW OF APPROACH

The following recommended nutrition standards have two major objectives. The first is to encourage the consumption of foods and beverages that are healthful for children, for example, fruits, vegetables, whole grains, and nonfat or low-fat dairy products. The second objective is to limit wherever possible, in all competitive foods and beverages offered at schools, food components that are not healthful when consumed in excess. Fats, sodium, added sugars, nonnutritive sweeteners, and caffeine were included.

To achieve these parallel aims, three categories of competitive foods and beverages for school-age children were defined. Tier 1 foods and beverages are desirable to encourage; Tier 2 foods and beverages do not exceed an acceptable level of total, saturated, and trans fat; sugars; and sodium; and finally, the third category includes foods and beverages that do not meet the standards described in the DGA and are not allowed. Other approaches were also considered, such as a single tier rather than two, and including half servings of Tier 1 foods per portion as packaged. However, the committee determined that the Tier system was preferable to achieve the goals of the Guiding Principles.

The intended outcome of the committee's recommendations is as follows:

• Tier 1 foods may be offered throughout the school day at all school levels, if school administrators elect to make competitive foods and beverages available.
• Tier 2 foods and beverages are available at limited times of the day at specified school levels.
• All other competitive foods are not made available during the school day or at after-school activities for students. These competive foods may be offered at certain after-school acitivities, particularly on occasions

such as school concerts or sporting events, when adults as well as students, are present.

HIERARCHY OF FOODS

To describe the standards, formal definitions of key concepts were developed. These include specific definitions of the hierarchy of competitive foods and beverages. This hierarchy is called Tier 1 and Tier 2 to classify competitive foods and beverages by their compliance with DGA recommendations. The committee evaluated the nutrient content of food items to determine whether they conform to the nutrition standards in this report based on the recommendations of the DGA.

Tier 1 Foods and Beverages

Tier 1 foods and beverages provide important health benefits that warrant encouraging consumption by school-age children, and do not exceed levels of certain nutrients and compounds that may be unhealthful for school-age children when consumed in excess.

Types of Foods and Beverages Included in Tier 1

These food and beverage types listed as "foods to encourage" are derived from those with a similar definition described in the DGA (DHHS/USDA, 2005):

- Fruits and vegetables
- 100-percent fruit and vegetable juices
- Whole-grain products
- Nonfat or low-fat dairy products

Other foods and beverages are included as Tier 1:

- Nuts and seeds (allowed as combination products as long as other nutrient standards are met; the fat content will not count against the total fat content of the product)
- Entrée items included in the National School Lunch and School Program (NSLP) and School Breakfast Program (SBP) sold à la carte or entrée items comparable in portion size, calories, and nutritional value to NSLP/SBP entrées
- Water

Fruits, vegetables, and whole grains Fruits, vegetables, and whole grains are Tier 1 foods because of the health benefits they provide. The DGA indicates that current evidence is sufficiently compelling to justify the use of a "Fruit, Vegetable, and Whole-Grain Focus" as a foundation for a healthful diet. Although the functions of individual nutrients, such as vitamins and minerals, are well understood, many of the interactions between nutrients and other components found in whole foods are not, and remain to be elucidated.

The following provide the foundation for the committee's designation:

• These foods are important sources of many of the nutrients identified in Chapter 2 as those in which children's diets tend to be deficient, including calcium, potassium, fiber, magnesium, and vitamin E.

• Although the exact mechanisms are not fully understood, extensive epidemiological evidence shows that intake of generous amounts of these food groups is associated with reduced risk of chronic disease.

• Fruits, vegetables, and whole grains are often lower-calorie alternatives to foods and beverages also high in fats, sugar, and sodium. Thus, increased consumption of fruits, vegetables, and whole grains may be useful to achieve and manage a healthy weight.

• Many 9- to 13-year-olds do not meet the DGA (DHHS/USDA, 2005) recommendations for fruit and vegetable consumption. For example, fewer than 4 percent of girls and about 1 percent of boys meet the recommendations; among older children, less than 1 percent of boys and 1.5 percent of girls ages 14 to 18 years meet current recommendations (Guenther et al., 2006).

• The DGA (DHHS/USDA, 2005) recommends that half of daily grain consumption, or about three servings per day, be eaten as whole grains. A serving is defined as an ounce-equivalent, that is, a quantity of food containing 1 ounce of grain: one slice of bread, 1 ounce of dry cereal, or 1/2 cup of cooked rice, pasta, or cereal. Consumption of the equivalent of at least three 1-ounce servings of whole grains each day is recommended to help reduce the risk of several chronic diseases, and to help with weight maintenance. However, the average intake of whole grains is currently less than one serving per day, with less than 10 percent of all Americans consuming three servings per day (Cleveland et al., 2000).

To qualify as Tier 1 products, each item must contain at least one serving of a fruit or vegetable, as defined by the U.S. Department of Agriculture (USDA) "MyPyramid" and/or one serving of whole grain, as discussed above. In the case of combination products, the product must contain an aggregate of at least one serving of qualifying ingredients (e.g., one-half serving of fruit plus one-half serving of whole grain). A smaller portion size is acceptable for younger children as long as the constitution of the whole food component does not change.

Tier 1 combination products can include additional ingredients that are consistent with the recommended nutrition standards. For example, a baked fruit bar containing one serving of fruit and made with refined white flour still qualifies as a Tier 1 food, based on its fruit content, although the use of whole grain would be even more desirable.

The form of a food may affect its healthfulness. For example, it is likely that an apple eaten raw, with the peel on, may be more nutritionally beneficial than a highly processed apple juice. Components of Tier 1 products should be kept as close to their natural state as can be achieved while maintaining palatability and affordability.

Tier 1 foods consist of the following:

• Fruits and vegetables offered as individual pieces (e.g., apples, pears, carrots) or as products as close as possible to their natural state (e.g., applesauce, dried fruit, diced pears). These products must meet all other nutrition standards as specified in the committee's criteria.

• Whole-grain products (e.g., bagels, crackers, whole-grain chips) provide at least one serving of whole grains per portion and meet all other nutrition standards in this report.

• Combination products may take many different forms and must meet the following standards:

—One portion of the product contains at least one serving of fruit, vegetable, or whole grain in any combination (e.g., ½ serving of fruit plus ½ serving of whole grain, or ⅔ serving of fruit and ⅓ serving of whole grain).

—The number of servings (or fractions) of fruit and vegetable, and grams of whole grains in one portion, is clearly labeled or otherwise identifiable.

—The product may contain ingredients in addition to the above quantities of fruits, vegetables, and whole grains (e.g., yogurt, cheese, refined grains, nuts and seeds), but must meet all other nutrition standards as recommended in this report. A special allowance is made for nuts and seeds when they occur in combination products.

• Nonfat and low-fat yogurts may be offered, provided they contain no more than 30 grams of total sugars per 8-ounce serving (see "Added sugars information" below).

Nuts and seeds The committee also supports the inclusion of nut and seed products in Tier 1, as long as the products meet other nutrition standards. In addition, the fat content of nuts and seeds will not count against the total fat content of combination products. In particular, nuts and seeds, like fruits and vegetables, are whole foods (see Chapter 2) with complex nutrient structures. Although less research is available on the benefits of nuts and seeds, compared to fruits and vegetables, it is reasonable to accept that they may offer many of the same nutritional advantages noted for fruits and vegetables. Nuts are also specifically mentioned in the DGA as a source of beneficial fats for children (DHHS/USDA, 2005).

Nuts and seeds are good sources of monounsaturated fatty acids (MUFAs) and polyunsaturated fatty acids (PUFAs), which are the types of fats that should make up most of the fat in the diet. Some PUFAs are essential for health—the body cannot synthesize them from other fats. Some nuts and seeds (e.g., flax, walnuts) are excellent sources of essential fatty acids; and sunflower seeds, almonds, and hazelnuts are good sources of vitamin E. In addition, nuts and seeds may contribute to the overall compositional complexity of the diets with benefits as yet undocumented. In conjunction with their nutrient density, nuts and seeds are also energy dense, however nut and seed snack products are often high in sodium, and could contribute to excessive caloric and sodium intake.

Nonfat and low-fat dairy products Nonfat and low-fat dairy products are Tier 1 foods because of the critical importance of calcium, particularly for adolescent girls for whom calcium consumption can have a critical impact on the likelihood of developing osteoporosis later in life. The DGA (DHHS/USDA, 2005) recommends that children 4 to 8 years of age consume 2 cups of milk per day and those 9 to 18 years of age consume 3 cups per day. Milk consumption among children and adolescents is currently below this level and has been declining over the past few decades (see Chapter 2).

Juice One hundred-percent fruit and vegetable juices are both included in Tier 1 for reasons previously discussed for whole fruits and vegetables, although juices provide less dietary fiber than whole fruits or vegetables. This recommendation follows the Report of the Dietary Guidelines Advisory Committee (DGAC) in classifying juices as contributing to the recommended servings for the fruits and vegetables group (DHHS/USDA, 2004).

Because of concerns about excess juice consumption leading to excess energy intake, as well as certain other health issues such as displacing other more nutrient-dense foods, both the DGAC (DHHS/USDA, 2004) and the American Academy of Pediatrics (AAP, 2001) recommend that juice intake be limited. Consistent with this, the maximum juice portion sizes recommended are 4 and 8 ounces in elementary/middle and high schools, respectively.

Components of Federally Reimbursable Meals Also Sold as À La Carte

As noted in Chapter 3, among the most popular competitive food and beverage items sold are entrée or side item foods and beverages, which are offered both in the reimbursable school meals and as individual à la carte items (e.g., fresh fruit and yogurt salad).

Evidence from the most recent USDA School Nutrition and Dietary Assessment (SNDA-II) supports this by reporting that the offerings of the NSLP and SBP are reasonably nutritious and are improving in quality over time.

The nutrient standards of the diet-based federally reimbursable school nutrition programs are not the same as those recommended in this report for individual competitive foods and beverages. However, the two sets of rules overlap, and the committee concluded that it is reasonable to include these NSLP/SBP items in the set of Tier 1 foods and beverages to be encouraged when competitive foods are offered in schools, if they meet the nutrient standards as defined in this report.

Tier 2 Foods and Beverages

Tier 2 foods and beverages (allowed after school in high schools) fall short of Tier 1 standards, but are still consistent with the nutritional recommendations of the DGA. One difference from this general definition of Tier 2 foods and beverages is that the committee proposes that, for high schools, nonnutritive-sweetened beverages containing less than 5 calories per serving are included in Tier 2, while use of nonnutritive sweeteners are not addressed in the DGA.

The reason for the committee's proposed standard is that these beverages may provide alternatives that can be useful in (1) providing additional dietary choices to high school students, reflecting their development and level of responsibility, and (2) helping these students limit caloric intake. The decision to include this exemption represented a complex weighting of several competing goals (for further discussion see Chapter 2).

Foods and Beverages Not to Be Sold as Competitive Foods and Beverages

Excluded from Tier 1 and Tier 2 foods and beverages are those that do not meet the DGA for total, saturated and trans fat, added sugars, and sodium. The standards for Tier 1, Tier 2, and à la carte foods and beverages are summarized in Table 5-1.

TABLE 5-1 Foods and Beverages That Meet Tier 1 and Tier 2 Standards

Foods	Beverages
Tier 1 for All Students	
Tier 1 foods are fruits, vegetables, whole grains, and related combination products* and nonfat and low-fat dairy that are limited to 200 calories or less per portion as packaged and	Tier 1 beverages are
• No more than 35 percent of total calories from fat	• Water without flavoring, additives, or carbonation
• Less than 10 percent of total calories from saturated fats	• Low-fat* and nonfat milk (in 8 oz. portions):
• Zero trans fat (≤ 0.5 g per serving)	—Lactose-free and soy beverages are included
• 35 percent or less of calories from total sugars, except for yogurt with no more than 30 g of total sugars, per 8-oz. portion as packaged	—Flavored milk with no more than 22 g of total sugars per 8-oz. portion
• Sodium content of 200 mg or less per portion as packaged	• 100 percent fruit juice in 4-oz. portion as packaged for elementary/middle school and 8 oz. (two portions) for high school
	• Caffeine-free, with the exception of trace amounts of naturally occurring caffeine substances
À la carte entrée items meet fat and sugar limits as listed above and**	
—Are National School Lunch Program (NSLP) menu items	
—Have a sodium content of 480 mg or less	
*Combination products must contain a total of one or more servings as packaged of fruit, vegetables, or whole-grain products per portion	*1-percent milk fat
**200-calorie limit does not apply; items cannot exceed calorie content of comparable NSLP entrée items	
Tier 2 for High School Students After School	
Tier 2 snack foods are those that do not exceed 200 calories per portion as packaged and	Tier 2 beverages are
• No more than 35 percent of total calories from fat	• Non-caffeinated, non-fortified beverages with less than 5 calories per portion as packaged (with or without nonnutritive sweeteners, carbonation, or flavoring)
• Less than 10 percent of total calories from saturated fats	
• Zero trans fat (≤ 0.5 g per portion)	
• 35 percent or less of calories from total sugars	
• Sodium content of 200 mg or less per portion as packaged	

Recommended Standards for Competitive Foods and Beverages Offered in Schools

The committee's Guiding Principles and the concept of Tier 1 and Tier 2 foods form the basis of its recommendations for nutrition standards for competitive foods offered in schools. These standards have two major objectives. The first is to encourage children to consume foods and beverages that are healthful—fruits, vegetables, whole grains, and nonfat or low-fat dairy products. The second objective is, wherever possible in all competitive foods and beverages offered at schools, to limit food components that are either not healthful when consumed at levels exceeding the DGA or fall outside DGA recommendations. Standards that contain specified ranges for fats, energy, added sugar, and sodium are the committee's best judgment derived from limited available evidence, and the rationale is explained in relevant portions of the text.

Dietary Fats

Standard 1: Snacks, foods, and beverages meet the following criteria for dietary fat per portion as packaged:

- No more than 35 percent of total calories from fat
- Less than 10 percent of total calories from saturated fats
- Zero trans fats

Rationale

Americans, including children, consume too much total dietary fat, especially saturated fats. Although some fat intake is needed to meet requirements for essential fatty acids and to utilize fat-soluble vitamins, fats are energy dense, and a high fat intake is a major contributor to the high caloric intake of overweight and obese individuals. Data are consistently strong that diets high in saturated fat are associated with increased risk for and higher rates of coronary heart disease. Like saturated fats, trans fats, found in hydrogenated oils, increase low-density lipoprotein (LDL) cholesterol; trans fats also decrease high-density lipoprotein (HDL) cholesterol. The DGA recommends 25 to 35 percent of calories from total fat for all individuals over 2 years of age. The recommended standard for school-age children (4–19 years of age), is the upper end of an acceptable range in the DGA (and in the Dietery Reference Intakes, or DRIs), and allows for greater flexibility in choices while remaining within acceptable limits for a dietary pattern.

Added Sugars

Standard 2: Snacks, foods, and beverages provide no more than 35 percent of calories from total sugars per portion as packaged.
Exceptions include

- 100-percent fruits and fruit juices in all forms without added sugars
- 100-percent vegetables and vegetable juices without added sugars
- Unflavored nonfat and low-fat milk and yogurt; flavored nonfat and low-fat milk with no more than 22 grams of total sugars per 8-ounce serving; and flavored nonfat and low-fat yogurt with no more than 30 grams of total sugars per 8-ounce serving

Rationale

Balancing food energy intake levels with energy expenditure is consistent with maintaining healthy weight. Sugars contain calories without substantial amounts of micronutrients. Limiting foods high in added sugars is recommended because of its association with increased calorie consumption and decreased intake of micronutrients. Decreases in micronutrient intake are strongest when added sugars exceed 25 percent of the total caloric intake.

Although the committee concluded that the ideal recommendation for added sugars would be one that limits them to no more than 25 percent or less of total calories, such a recommendation for sugars could not be operationalized at this time because manufacturers are not required to list added sugars as part of the nutrition facts panel. The committee established the interim recommendation of 35 percent of calories from total sugars (with exceptions noted above) versus added sugars, because the total sugars information is part of the nutrition facts panel.

A standard based on calories versus one based on weight is a reasonable calculation and will allow for a greater variety of products, such as cereals and granola bars, to be provided. Many of these products are important contributors of folate, vitamins A and C, iron, and zinc in children's diets. It should be noted that the committee considered setting the added sugars limit at 10 percent for individual foods, but it was determined that a 25 percent limit, with the exception of dairy products, would be more easily achieved, while still contributing to improvement in the eating patterns of school-age children.

Recently, the contribution of added sugars from soft drinks, fruitades, and other sweetened fruit drinks to the total intake of added sugars in children's diets ranged from 35 to more than 50 percent. Other recommendations from the committee will eliminate all non-dairy beverages with added sugars from schools, thus reducing sugar consumption to more closely align with levels recommended by the World Health Organization (WHO, 2003) (see Chapter 2).

As noted above, the recommendation of 35 percent of calories from total sugars (with exceptions noted above) is viewed by the committee as an interim recommendation until added sugars information is more readily available to school foodservice operators.

Added sugars information Ultimately, the committee urges USDA and school foodservice operators to require that food manufacturers selling their products to schools make information regarding added sugars available (see Action 2). To this end, USDA may want to consider updating regulations for the Child Nutrition (CN) Labeling Program, requiring manufacturers to provide added sugars information. This would require the list of products that are now eligible for CN labeling to be expanded (the current list includes only meat/meat alternate, and minimum 50-percent juice products). Alternatively, USDA may want to establish guidelines for snacks and beverages that include requiring manufacturers to provide added sugars information as part of the product nutrient profile. When added sugars information is provided, the committee recommends that products contain no more than 25 percent of calories as added sugars.

Rationale for the fruit and vegetable exception Although fruits and vegetables are listed as an exception, the exception does not indicate that the sugars limit is raised. Rather, it takes into consideration the high natural sugar content of fruits (and some vegetables)—fresh, juiced, frozen, canned, and dried—and recognizes the DGA recommendation calling for Americans to consume more fruits and vegetables in all forms. This is especially important for children, many of whom do not meet DGA recommendations for fruits and vegetables. Because foodservice operators will be able to determine if sugars are added through the ingredient panel on juiced, canned, frozen, and dried fruit and vegetable products, the exception merely allows all forms of fruits and vegetables—with no added sugars—to be provided and promoted.

Rationale for the dairy product exception Exceptions for dairy products are included for a number of reasons. Dietary intake of calcium-rich foods and beverages is very important throughout life, and especially important in late childhood and adolescence when the rate of bone calcium accretion is highest as reflected in the increased DRI for calcium between the ages of 9 and 18 years. However, many dairy products, such as fruit-flavored yogurt, that are popular among school-age children contain added sugars in excess of 25 percent of calories, and total sugars in excess of 35 percent of calories. To avoid elimination of these dairy products on the basis of their sugars content, the committee has made an exception to the added sugars limit. In setting the proposed higher standards for dairy products, the committee attempted to set limits that are attainable while maintaining product palatability, and reducing intake of added sugars from these products. The total sugars limit for flavored milk, set at 22 grams per 8-ounce serving, will allow for about 10 grams of added sugars because the naturally occurring sugar content in nonfat and low-fat milk is about 12 grams (USDA, 2005). The total sugars limit for flavored yogurt, set at 30 grams per 8-ounce serving, will allow for about 12 grams of added sugars because the naturally occurring sugars content in nonfat and low-fat yogurt is about 18 grams (USDA, 2005). In making its recommendations, the committee is mindful of the positive efforts of some states and school districts, sometimes working together with the dairy industry, to develop dairy products lower in added sugars.

Calorie Limits

Standard 3: Snack items are 200 calories or less per portion as packaged and à la carte entrée items do not exceed calorie limits on comparable NSLP items. For à la carte entrée items, the 200-calorie limit does not apply and does not exceed the calorie content of comparable NSLP entrée items.

Rationale

Most U.S. children consume at least one snack per day, consuming nearly one quarter of their dietary energy intake as snacks. Energy intake should be commensurate with energy expenditure in order to achieve energy balance and avoid overweight and obesity. Unhealthy weight gain may develop over time from a relatively small daily excess of calories consumed, the energy density of foods being higher for snacks compared to meals. In accordance with estimates of energy needs and accounting for physical activity levels, the committee calculated that approximately 91 percent of daily energy intake would be consumed as meals, leaving no more than 9 percent of total daily energy intake for discretionary energy consumption from snacks (see discussion in Chapter 2). The committee's judgment is that a 200-calorie maximum limit per portion for snacks may be high for some children, but it is assumed that variations in other daily caloric intake will compensate for shortfalls or excesses.

Furthermore, à la carte entrée items should not provide more calories or larger portion sizes than the comparable NSLP entrée items they may replace. The standard is established for whole servings rather than half servings because, in the committee's judgment, a whole serving of fruit, vegetable, or whole grain per portion would contribute to the goal of helping school-age children meet DGA recommendations in a portion size that food manufacturers can achieve in formulating new products.

Sodium

Standard 4: Snack items meet a sodium content limit of 200 mg or less per portion as packaged or 480 mg or less per entrée portion as served for à la carte.

Rationale

Although sodium is an essential mineral, it is widely overconsumed. Research evidence in adult human subjects strongly supports an association between salt intake and increased blood pressure, although similar associations in children and adolescents are not as well-documented.

The exception to this recommendation for entrée items purchased à la carte reflects the fact that they generally represent greater portion sizes than the recommended calorie limit for snacks would allow; these entrée items are components of meals that meet USDA school meal nutrition standards and the FDA maximum sodium levels allowed for foods labeled as "healthy." Their inclusion allows greater flexibility for students with greater energy needs.

Nonnutritive Sweeteners

Standard 5: Beverages containing nonnutritive sweeteners are only allowed in high schools after the end of the school day.

Factors Considered for Use of Nonnutritive Sweeteners

In consideration of nonnutritive sweeteners in competitive foods and beverages for school-age children, four related topics were evaluated: safety of nonnutritive sweeteners in children; displacement effect of intake of foods and beverages with nonnutritive sweeteners on intake of other foods and beverages to be encouraged (fruits, vegetables, whole grains, and nonfat or low-fat dairy products); efficacy of intake of foods and beverages containing nonnutritive sweeteners to contribute to maintaining a healthy weight in children; and the role of choice and necessity in the use of nonnutritive sweeteners in beverages and foods.

Safety The Food and Drug Administration (FDA) sets safety standards for food additives, including nonnutritive sweeteners. Those that are approved for use have been evaluated extensively and have met FDA safety standards. Although safety standards are in place for food additives, there is still uncertainty, particularly about long-term use and about low-level exposure effects on health and development in children.

Displacement of foods and beverages to be encouraged Nonnutritive-sweetened beverages may be chosen instead of nutrient-dense beverages. Nutrient displacement occurs when a beverage or food of lesser nutritional value is substituted for one of greater nutritional value, resulting in reduced intake of nutrients.

Efficacy of nonnutritive sweeteners for weight control The DGA states that reduction of calorie intake is important in weight control. Nonnutritive sweeteners are used to replace sugars in foods and beverages and provide lower calorie choices to consumers.

Choice and necessity Beverages that meet Tier 2 standards and have no caloric contribution increase the number of choices. Snack foods that meet Tier 1 and 2 requirements can meet calorie limits by substituting nonnutritive sweeteners for sugars. These additional choices may be useful for those who wish to control or maintain body weight; however, the use of nonnutritive sweeteners to provide lower calorie foods and beverages is not necessary to achieve weight control. The committee considered these issues in the context of developmental and social skills of school-age children and the public health concern of childhood obesity.

Rationale for Nonnutritive-Sweetened Beverages

Safety The FDA sets a safety standard for foods or food additives, regulated by the Federal Food, Drug, and Cosmetic Act, of "a reasonable certainty of no harm." Prior to their approval for use, the FDA reviewed numerous safety studies on nonnutritive sweeteners in current use and has not, to date, found an associated safety risk. There is, however, a paucity of evidence on long-term health effects in humans from nonnutritive sweeteners, particularly exposure initiated in childhood.

Displacement Soft drinks do not provide nutrients identified as lacking in the diets of U.S. children. These beverages could, if offered during the school day, displace more nutrient-rich products, such as nonfat and low-fat milk or 100-percent juice. The committee determined this was less of a consideration outside meal times, when milk and juice consumption is believed to be relatively low. The committee found no evidence to evaluate the impact of nonnutritive-sweetened products to increase the consumption of foods and beverages to be encouraged (fruits, vegetables, whole grains, and nonfat or low-fat dairy products).

Efficacy Evidence shows that diets that use nonnutritive-sweetened products can aid in weight loss and/or maintenance (i.e., weight control) in obese adult women. In these studies, nonnutritive sweeteners were generally consumed in beverages. No evidence is available to evaluate the efficacy of nonnutritive-sweetened foods for weight control. Preliminary evidence from a pilot study in adolescents indicated that replacing sugar-sweetened beverages with nonnutritive-sweetened beverages could help obese adolescents with weight control.

Nonnutritive-sweetened beverages provide low-calorie choices that may effectively contribute to weight control. High school-age students may be better able to discriminate among more or less healthful choices and better prepared to make informed, individually appropriate beverage choices than younger school-age children.

Necessity Although the DGA and the DGAC acknowledged that obesity is a major public health concern, they remained silent on the use of nonnutritive sweeteners as part of the strategy to maintain a healthy weight in Americans, including school-age children. The DGAC literature review did not include a review of the efficacy of nonnutritive sweeteners for weight loss and weight maintenance and the DGA did not address nonnutritive sweeteners as part of the strategy to maintain a healthy weight in Americans, including school-age children. The DGA does state that reduction of caloric intake is important in weight control; thus use of nonnutritive sweeteners could be a weight control strategy for some populations, but are not necessary to achieve this goal.

Conclusion Based on the lack of evidence to evaluate efficacy and with an intention to avoid complexity of standards across age groups and times of day, the committee took a cautious approach in its recommendations and determined that nonnutritive sweeteners are limited to beverages for high school students after school, thus avoiding competition with and potential displacement of nutrient-rich products as part of school meals and snacks.

Rationale on Nonnutritive-Sweetened Foods

Because of the uncertainties and limitations in evidence, especially concerning the safety and benefits for weight control, the committee does not recommend a standard for nonnutritive sweeteners in foods.

Safety Nonnutritive sweeteners have been evaluated and meet the safety standards set by FDA. However, there is no long-term evidence on the safety of nonnutritive sweeteners when consumption begins in early childhood and in relation to a broader range of health and developmental outcomes. The committee considered this in light of the limitations in testing and the lack of evidence concerning the benefits or necessity for use of nonnutritive sweeteners in foods.

Efficacy Based on the energy balance principle, nonnutritive sweeteners in foods might provide a tool for weight management; however, studies to test this concept have not been conducted in children and the complexities of nonnutritive sweeteners and appetite have not been studied in this age group. Moreover, improving diet and maintenance of healthy weight in children does not require foods with nonnutritive sweeteners. There was a concern that children may not be able to distinguish between a nonnutritive sweetened food and a similar full-calorie food, which might encourage unintentional overconsumption of calories.

Necessity Although nonnutritive sweeteners may increase palatability, thereby increasing the consumption of healthful foods, the potential increase in consumption may not be sufficient reason to include nonnutritive sweeteners in foods.

Displacement Displacement was not an important issue for nonnutritive sweeteners in foods that otherwise meet the recommended standards.

Conclusion Given these uncertainties and limitations, research is needed, particularly on safety and efficacy.

Caffeine

Standard 6: Foods and beverages are caffeine free, with the exception of trace amounts of naturally occurring caffeine-related substances.

Rationale

The evidence for adverse health effects, other than physical dependency and withdrawal from caffeine consumption, varies in severity of effects and consistency of results among studies (see discussion in Chapter 2) except for physical dependency and withdrawal symptoms. Tolerance and dependence on caffeine have been identified in all ages, including school-age children, and withdrawal from regular caffeine intake is followed by generally mild effects such as moodiness, headache, and shakiness.

Although there may be some benefits associated with caffeine consumption among adults (see Chapter 2), the committee did not support offering products containing significant amounts of caffeine for school-age children because of the potential for adverse effects, including physical dependency and withdrawal (described in Chapter 2). Thus the committee judged that caffeine in significant quantities has no place in foods and beverages offered in schools. The committee recognized that some foods and beverages contain trace amounts of naturally occurring caffeine and related substances. The intent of the committee was not to exclude such foods or beverages if the amounts of caffeine consumed are small and the product otherwise complies with the recommended nutrition standards.

Foods and Beverages Offered in Schools

Standard 7: Foods and beverages offered during the school day are limited to those in Tier 1.

Rationale

Tier 1 foods and beverages have particular attributes making them "foods and beverages to encourage." Thus it is appropriate to make them available as snacks throughout the school day and as à la carte items during school meal periods. As discussed in Chapter 2, the evidence supports the use of Tier 1 foods to

- increase the current consumption of fruits, vegetables, and whole grains by school-age children;
- increase consumption of calcium-rich foods and beverages;
- set standards for à la carte entrées that meet NSLP requirements or the recommended standards herein; and
- reinforce innovation by industry to create food and dairy products more consistent with the DGA, thereby increasing healthful food choices for school-age children.

The committee concludes that policies encouraging the sale of fruit-, vegetable-, and whole grain-based foods and nonfat or low-fat dairy products in à la carte lines, vending machines, school stores, snack bars, fundraisers, and other venues will be nutritionally beneficial.

Standard 8: Plain, potable water is available throughout the school day at no cost to students.

Rationale

Water is essential to health, and is naturally calorie-free with few known negative health consequences. Either tap or bottled water or water from fountains or other sources represents a safe, desirable way of maintaining hydration during the school day, and is therefore included as a Tier 1 beverage. The committee's interpretation of limited available evidence is that carbonated water, fortified water, flavored water, and similar products are excluded during the school day, because such products are associated with displacement of more healthful beverages (see Chapter 2), they are unneccessary for hydration purposes, and the increasing number of products increases the difficulty of making clear distinctions among them. In addition, if flavored or fortified waters are included, they may serve, in the committee's judgment, as implicit encouragement to produce more foods with nonnutritive components for children at the expense of the more heathful fruits, vegetables, whole grains, and nonfat and low-fat dairy products.

Standard 9: Sports drinks are not available in the school setting except when provided by the school for student athletes participating in sport programs involving vigorous activity of more than one hour's duration.

Rationale

The committee concluded that, in most contexts, sports drinks are equivalent to flavored water, and because of their high sugar content it is appropriate that they be excluded from both Tier 1 and 2 beverages. However, for students engaged in prolonged, vigorous activities on hot days, evidence suggests sports drinks are useful for facilitating hydration, providing energy, and replacing electrolytes. The committee's recommended standard is consistent with conclusions of expert panels who considered this issue in adults. The committee suggests that the individual athletic coach determine whether sports drinks are made available to student athletes under allowable conditions to maintain hydration.

Standard 10: Foods and beverages are not used as rewards or discipline for academic performance or behavior.

Rationale

Some schools have reported the use of foods and beverages as an aid in managing behavior. The committee has determined that such use of foods in schools is inappropriate; thus to avoid establishing an emotional connection between foods and beverages and acomplishment, they should not be allowed.

Standard 11: Minimize marketing of Tier 2 foods and beverages in the high school setting by

• locating Tier 2 food and beverage distribution in low student traffic areas; and
• ensuring that the exterior of vending machines does not depict commercial products or logos or suggest that consumption of vended items conveys a health or social benefit.

Rationale

The presence in some high schools of vending machines used to sell Tier 2 foods and beverages after school leaves open a marketing opportunity for industry to promote their products during the regular school day, even if these vending machines are only turned on at the end of the regular school day. In making this recommendation, the committee concurs with the recommendations of the recent Institute of Medicine report on food and beverage marketing to children.

Foods and Beverages Offered in the After-School Setting

Standard 12: Tier 1 snack items are allowed after school for student activities for elementary and middle schools. Tier 1 and 2 snacks are allowed after school for high school.

Defining end of the regular school day Implementing the above concept will require that schools develop an operational definition of the time when the regular school day ends for high school. The committee has elected to leave the determination of the end of the school day to the local principal or other school administrator familiar with local circumstances. Some high schools may wish to define the end of the school day as the end of classes. This would make Tier 2 foods available to students as snacks while they are leaving school; other schools may wish to limit departing students to the most healthy foods by enabling the availability of only Tier 2 foods, after most students have left campus—perhaps one-half hour after the last class has ended. Avoiding congestion as students seek to board buses or leave through a limited number of exits may be additional factors to consider.

Rationale

The committee's recommended standard applies specifically to after-school activities that are attended mainly by students and thus represent an extension of the regular school day. Many school-related activities take place in the late afternoon and evening and involve both students and adults or, in some instances, mainly adults. These include interscholastic sporting events, back-to-school nights, parent-teacher assocation meetings, and use of the school for adult activities such as adult athletic leagues.

Some students remain on the campus and proceed directly to their after-school activities, while others leave campus and return for these activities. Some food consumed during the after-school period is provided by the school, while in other cases it is provided by students or others.

Given that high school students are often expected to handle more responsibility, it is appropriate to give them more choice in the less formal environment after the school day. Tier 2 foods and beverages provide for an expanded variety while still maintaining nutrition standards.

Standard 13: For on-campus fund-raising activities during the school day, Tier 1 foods and beverages are allowed for elementary, middle, and high schools. Tier 2 foods and beverages are allowed for high schools after school. For evening and community activities that include adults, Tier 1 and 2 foods and beverages are encouraged.

Rationale

Fund-raisers that include the use of foods and beverages should emphasize nutritious choices such as fruits or juices, vegetables, nuts, grain products, and nonfat and low-fat dairy products. The committee recognizes that there are many activities that involve both students and adults or, in some instances, mainly adults. These include interscholastic sport events, back-to-school nights, parent-teacher association meetings, and use of the school for specifically adult activities such as athletic leagues. The committee recognizes that attempting to regulate foods and beverages sold for fund-raising or offered at evening events attended by both students and adults is not practical and may not be desirable. However, the committee urges that when foods and beverages are included in such activities they be limited to items that meet Tier 1 and 2 standards.

Actions for the Implementation of Nutrition Standards in Schools

Action 1: Appropriate policy-making bodies ensure that recommendations are fully adopted by providing

- regulatory guidance to federal, state, and local authorities;
- designated responsibility for overall coordination and oversight to federal, state, and local authorities; and
- performance-based guidelines and technical and financial support to schools or school districts, as needed.

Rationale

Policy changes will be required to implement these recommendations. These changes can be made at the local (school or school district) level, at the state level, or at the national level, using various combinations of policy guidance, regulations, legislation, etc. To implement these recommendations successfully, an agency with authority and capacity must be designated to coordinate and monitor the implementation. In addition, most potential implementing agencies will need assistance—in the form of information, advice, model strategies, and, in some cases, funding. The committee used this approach because not all schools require technical and financial support and because the type and amount of support needed will vary across districts.

Action 2: Appropriate federal agencies engage with the food industry to

- establish a user-friendly identification system for Tier 1 and 2 snacks, foods, and beverages that meet the standards per portion as packaged; and
- provide specific guidance for whole-grain products and combination products that contain fruits, vegetables, and whole grains.

Rationale

Implementing the standards recommended in this report for Tier 1 and Tier 2 foods and beverages and on other issues regarding food content will be accomplished only with coordination and cooperation among federal agencies and the food industry. If school food service operators are to identify and evaluate foods and beverages that meet certain standards, they will need detailed product information from manufacturers. Product information that is currently available to foodservice operators is not always sufficient to ensure that products meet nutrition standards. For example, although some product information is readily available, such as total and saturated fat and sodium, other information, such as added sugars, whole-grain status, and fruit content, may be more difficult to determine. The committee urges appropriate federal agencies and food manufacturers to develop an identification system that will enable school foodservice operators to easily evaluate whether a product meets certain standards. The Centers for Disease Control and Prevention and the Produce for Better Health Foundation "Products Promotable" guidelines are excellent examples of federal agencies working with the private sector to determine what fruit and vegetable products can bear the 5-A-Day logo. The committee recommends a similar approach that will require coordination among appropriate federal agencies as well as the private sector to establish a system to identify Tier 1 and Tier 2 foods as defined by the committee.

The committee recognizes that the development of an identification system is a longer term goal. In the interim, the committee has provided information on areas such as whole grains and added sugars to assist stakeholders in implementing the recommendations in the short term.

CONCLUSION

The federally reimbursable school nutrition programs traditionally have been an important means for ensuring that students have daily access to fruits, vegetables, whole-grain-based products, and nonfat or low-fat dairy products during the school day. The committee's view is that these programs should be the main source of nutrition provided at school. However, the committee also recognizes that there is an increasing number of opportunities for students to eat and drink, including à la carte services, vending machines, school stores, snack bars, concession stands, classroom or school celebrations, achievement rewards, after-school programs, and other venues. Thus schools are encouraged to limit such additional opportunities for students to eat and drink, but when they do arise in school, they should be used to encourage greater daily consumption of fruits, vegetables, whole grains, and nonfat or low-fat dairy products.

The committee also acknowledges that implementing new standards for competitive foods offered in schools will incur a transition phase and that offering a competitive food program is elective, and additional costs likely will be passed on to purchasers. However, the committee's reasoning is that increased market response with greater product availability will help diminish resistance to change.

The recommendations in this report are intended to ensure that offerings in these venues are consistent with the DGA and, in particular, to help children and adolescents meet the guidelines for consumption of fruits, vegetables, whole grains, and nonfat or low-fat dairy products.

6

Next Steps

IMPLEMENTATION OF SCHOOL STANDARDS: EVALUATING PROGRESS AND IMPACT

The recommended nutrition standards are one of several elements of a school nutrition policy that could significantly improve the nutritional quality of the foods available, promoted, and consumed in schools. To be effective, these standards must be implemented by a wide range of organizations and individuals: they must understand what is expected of them, and will need resources and support. A system is needed to track progress, resolve bottlenecks in implementation, and evaluate both the implementation and documentation and the resulting changes. While proposing a complete implementation and evaluation plan is beyond the scope of this committee, this chapter provides a framework and a set of benchmarks on which such a plan can be developed.

A Framework for Implementation

One way to identify the implementation requirements and the elements that should be tracked over time is to focus on the major steps needed from the time of the report release until changes in the diets of children during the school day have been established. Box 6-1 identifies four steps: awareness and understanding by diverse organizations; stakeholders decisions to implement the recommended nutrition standards by these organizations; changes in food and beverage availability in schools; and changes in the

**BOX 6-1
Key Elements for Success**

1. Awareness and understanding of the standards by personnel in schools, school boards, school district administrators, parents, students, health professionals and child advocates, state agencies, state boards of education and legislatures, Congress, the U.S. Department of Agriculture, the U.S. Department of Health and Human Services, the U.S. Department of Education, food and beverage industry, and vendors.
2. Actions taken to implement nutrition standards by those same personnel, potentially including
   - Supportive legislation at federal,state, and/or local levels
   - Supportive regulations issued by federal, state, and/or local agencies
   - Technical and financial support as needed
   - Incorporation of standards into school wellness policies
   - Development of food and beverage products that meet standards
3. Changes in food availability in schools, including
   - Products offered in à la carte, in vending machines, stores, and snack bars consistent with the standards
   - Products used in celebrations, fundraising, and after-school activities consistent with the standards
4. Changes in children's food and beverage sources and intake during the extended school day, including
   - Improved product profile (e.g., servings of food groups, types of beverages, etc.)
   - Improved nutrient composition of children's diets

dietary intake of children during the school day. Each of these is elaborated upon below, including specific suggestions for implementation and tracking of progress over time.

Awareness and Understanding of Standards

Awareness and understanding of the standards by personnel in schools, school boards, school district administrators, state agencies, state boards of education and legislatures, Congress, the U.S. Department of Agriculture (USDA), the U.S. Department of Health and Human Services (DHHS), food and beverage industry and vendors, as well as health professionals, child advocates, parents, and children are essential to implementation.

In recent years, many schools and local, state, and federal legislatures, as well as other agencies, have implemented a variety of model nutrition standards. The first step, therefore, is for the committee's recommendations to be disseminated and compared to current standards. In many cases, this may be a complex process because of the level of detail involved and investments already made in the current standards. In order for dissemination to be effectively carried out, states and school districts must harmonize their current standards with the new standards, to the greatest extent possible. Doing so will simplify many aspects of the on-going implementation, enforcement, and evaluation of nutrition standards and encourage industry to develop healthful products for the school setting. For example, making the recommendations (and simplified tools/resources based on them) available to the full range of school personnel will facilitate discussion of the recommendations at federal, state, and local levels, as well as school- and community-level promotional activities and training of local school staff.

Decisions and Actions

The second key element for success comprises positive decisions and actions taken to implement the standards, including

- supportive legislation at federal, state, and/or local levels;
- supportive regulations issued by federal, state, and/or local agencies;
- incorporation of standards into school wellness policies; and
- development of food and beverage products that meet the standards.

Until recently, foods and beverages served outside the federally reimbursable school nutrition programs have been largely unregulated in school settings. To be effective, the committee's recommendations will require a wide range of actions by legislatures, school boards, schools, government agencies, nonprofit organizations, and the food industry.

Taking steps to ensure that model nutrition standards and model school policies, as produced by many organizations in recent years, harmonize with the committee's recommended standards to the greatest extent possible will facilitate implementation and avoid confusion. By collaborating with the food and beverage industry, federal agencies will formalize criteria and labels for products for the school setting; develop similar criteria for whole-grain products; develop consistent criteria for combination products; and identify the amount of added sugars on the nutrition facts panel on labels as recommended in Chapter 5.

Changes in Food Availability

Positive changes in food and beverage availability and practices in schools include

- products offered à la carte and via vending machines, stores, and snack bars are consistent with the recommended standards; and
- products used in celebrations, fund-raising, and after-school activities are consistent with the standards.

While many of the foregoing identify decisions and actions needed at the state and federal levels, the success with which the recommended standards are translated into improved diets for school-age children depends on the ability and willingness of schools and school districts to implement them. Actions that facilitate this process are discussed below.

A responsible party such as the school wellness policy administrator may assume the task of ensuring compliance with nutrition standards. This work may be facilitated by the development of federal or state programs such as a Nutrition-Friendly Schools Initiative to encourage compliance and certify those schools that have fully complied with the recommended nutrition standards. Compliance can be verified and progress assessed by health educators, local health departments, or other outside stakeholders with similar expertise. In addition, schools might seek assistance from relevant state agencies, Centers for Disease Control and Prevention (CDC) staff, USDA regional offices, and qualified local organizations and agencies. Such assistance and collaboration would be greatly facilitated if state and federal agencies specifically earmarked funds for this purpose.

Changes in Food Sources

Positive changes in the food and beverage sources during the extended school day, including reformulating products to comply with the recommended standards and improving the nutrient composition of school-age children's diets, are the expected outcomes from implementation of the recommended nutrition standards. However, to ensure the success of the intended outcomes, it is important that benchmarking become a part of the implementation process.

Tracking Progress

One of the committee's assigned tasks was to develop benchmarks to guide future evaluation studies of the application of the recommended standards. In this report, the term "benchmarks" refers to the key elements of standards implementation and impact that would be most useful to evaluate.

The committee anticipates that the potential impact of the standards will be carefully considered by school districts, researchers from a number of related disciplines, and government agencies at the state and federal levels. Evaluation at the local level may enable school districts to document successes and to identify potential problems and devise solutions. Broader evaluation at the state and federal levels, and evaluations that may be more scientifically rigorous, will help to inform local, state, and national policy action on the recommended nutrition standards for schools. The evaluation process can be as simple as the development of a descriptive assessment checklist for key stakeholders in local school districts, or as complex as a meticulous pre- and post-intervention appraisal that is conducted as part of university research or as part of a broader evaluation at the state or federal level.

School districts, states, stakeholder organizations, and researchers may wish to discuss the potential for these evaluation options at the time that they plan the implementation of the new policies. It is advisable to examine the impact of the standards after they have been in place for at least one school year.

Ease and Extent of Nutrition Standards Adoption

In order for the recommended nutrition standards to be adopted, key decision-makers must be informed of the policy and understand its contents and likely outcomes. These decision-makers include some or all of the following individuals and groups: school personnel, especially those responsible for food acquisition and preparation; parents and parent organizations; school boards; school district administrators; state agencies and legislatures; key members of Congress and their staffs; federal agencies, especially USDA and CDC; and food and beverage producers and vendors. Important benchmarks to consider are the breadth and depth of the awareness and understanding of the nutrition standards by stakeholders and policymakers, and the extent to which the full policy is adopted and accepted. Key issues that might be examined include the use of the specific standards for foods and beverages; place-and-time rules; determination of whether the standards were used according to age group; observations on the practicality/impracticality of various aspects of the policy; and views on policy implementation barriers at the district or school level.

Other related questions may include, How well accepted is the policy among students (at different ages), parents, teachers, and the broader community? How are policies monitored and by whom? How well enforced is the policy in the day-to-day world of school? What are the specific enforcement issues, if any? What school-related factors explain the ease or difficulty of change?

Other benchmarks may include cataloging decisions at all levels of government that implement the recommended nutrition standards. Appropriate questions to consider are the following:

• Were new regulations or policies to implement part or all of these standards issued by local, state, or federal agencies?

• Was legislation requiring part or all of these nutrition standards adopted at the local, state, or federal levels?

The federally mandated local wellness policies and CDC school health program promotion initiatives both provide an excellent opportunity for school districts to set nutrition standards that only allow the offering of healthy foods and beverages. Were these standards incorporated in part or in full in local or state school wellness policies, or as part of the comprehensive coordinated school health programs recommended by CDC?

Response of Food Producers, Manufacturers, and Vendors

In order for the recommended nutrition standards to be successful, food producers, manufacturers, and vendors must supply the amounts, kinds, and forms of the fruits, vegetables, whole grains, and nonfat and low-fat dairy products needed. Manufacturers and vendors are the source of fruits, vegetables, and whole-grain and combination products that meet the recommended standards. Therefore, in some cases, foods and beverages may need to be reformulated or uniformly portion-packaged to comply with these standards. Entirely new products may also be developed. Examining whether those manufacturers that supply foods and beverages to schools are willing to match product offerings to schools' needs under the new standards is the role of evaluators of the implementation of the standards.

Moreover, it will be important to assess and recognize whether food and beverage providers of all types engage in any innovative marketing practices in schools to promote the healthful foods and beverages offered under the new nutrition standards. A related issue of interest will be whether local producers involved in "farm-to-school" efforts are able to take advantage of the changes in the nutrition standards to incorporate local produce and other products into the foods and beverages offered in the school setting.

Foods and Beverages Available in Schools

The standards cover foods and beverages offered à la carte, in vending machines, in student stores, and in snack bars, as well as those used in celebrations, in fund-raising, and during after-school activities. An examination of the actual foods and beverages available to students of different ages, in different school venues, and at different times of day will be an essential benchmark to determine if the standards change food availability in a positive way if new products are introduced that violate the spirit of the standards, or if "black marketing" of foods and beverages by students becomes a common practice.

Impact on Children's Diets

The ultimate goal of the recommended nutrition standards is to contribute positively to the nutritional quality and healthfulness of diets of school-age children and to the food habits they develop. Benchmarks in this area will include whether changes in the foods and beverages consumed during the school day and improvements in nutritional intake at school occurred.

For example:

•   Are children more likely to consume federally reimbursable school breakfasts and lunches and after school-snacks?
•   Are there changes in à la carte or vending sales or in the amounts and kinds of food purchased off campus or brought from home?
•   Do children consume increased numbers of servings of fruits, vegetables, nonfat and low-fat dairy products, and whole grains as a result of the implementation of these standards?
•   Do children consume less total, saturated, and trans fat; sodium and added sugar; and more fiber? Do they consume more water and fewer soft drinks?
•   Is excess caloric intake reduced as a result of the implementation of the standards?
•   Is there a significant increase in intakes of nutrients of concern?

In addition to the above, it will be useful for studies to examine whether the overall dietary intakes of children and/or the distributions of body mass indexes are affected positively by these changes. The tracking of these outcomes at local and state levels may also be useful for overall monitoring and community awareness purposes. However, users of such data must bear in mind that such outcomes reflect a much wider set of behavioral and environmental factors at home and in the community, and are not to be expected to change merely in response to improvements in the school food environment. Positive changes in dietary intake have been shown to improve health. However, in evaluating the impact of the standards, the general focus should be on whether dietary intake has changed as a result of differences in the kinds of foods and beverages made available during the school day.

Finally, it would be helpful to know whether there is an overall impact on those students who were most likely to consume competitive foods and beverages before the implementation of the recommended nutrition standards. This information will help in determining if changes in the kinds of offerings lead to greater improvements in their nutritional intake at school and if there was a spillover effect on their food attitudes or preferences beyond the school day.

Impact on School Operations and Finances

Major changes in one aspect of school operations can have related effects on other aspects of the school—positive and negative, expected and unexpected. It will be useful to examine what these effects may be. One is the potential impact on the overall school budget and on school food service revenues. Are revenues lost or gained, and in which areas of the budget? What are the impacts of these changes, and, in the case of lost revenue, if any, what changes have been made to reverse or adjust to the loss? Implementation of the recommended standards probably will influence other aspects of school operations, and these changes also could be examined and reported as part of the benchmarking process.

Programs That Track Progress

Examples of programs that track the progress of evaluation activities once they are put into practice include the CDC Youth Risk Behavior Surveillance System (YRBSS) and School Physical Activity and Nutrition (SPAN) survey. The YRBSS gathers data on six categories of priority health-risk behaviors among children and young adults, including unhealthy dietary behaviors, and physical inactivity. The YRBSS also monitors general health status and the prevalence of overweight and asthma in children and adolescents. The program includes a national school-based survey conducted by CDC and state and local school-based surveys conducted by state and local education and health agencies. Examples of ways that the national YRBSS data are used by CDC and other federal agencies include assessing trends in priority health-risk behaviors among high school students, and monitoring progress toward achieving fifteen *Healthy People 2010* health objectives. State and local agencies and nongovernmental organizations use YRBSS data to set school health and health promotion program goals, such as wellness policies; support modification of school health curricula programs; support new legislation and policies that promote health; and seek funding for new initiatives.

The SPAN survey was developed to assess nutrition behaviors, attitudes and knowledge, and physical activity behaviors among 4th, 8th, and 11th grade students. Example applications of the SPAN survey include SPAN 2000–2002 and 2004–2005 studies, the Houston-Harris County STEPS Consortium, the Travis County CATCH program, and Robert Wood Johnson Foundation projects. These programs illustrate how the benchmarks identified in this report could be incorporated into federal, state, and local systems to track the progress or outcomes from implementation of the recommended standards and actions.

SOME FINAL THOUGHTS

Although there are uncertainties about the optimal implementation process of the recommended nutrition standards, and their ultimate impact on the potential outcomes described in this chapter, the committee is confident that implementation will contribute greatly to an overall healthful eating environment in U.S. schools. Already, there are many success stories from schools, school districts, and states that have implemented standards similar to the ones proposed by the committee. Enhanced collaboration among the many affected groups, with sharing of different implementation strategies and outcome data, will provide guidance for ongoing and future efforts to improve the dietary intake and food habits of U.S. children.

7

References

CHAPTER 1

Cullen KW, Zakeri I. 2004. Fruits, vegetables, milk, and sweetened beverages consumption and access to à la carte/snack bar meals at school. *Am J Public Health* 94(3):463–467.

DHHS (U.S. Department of Health and Human Services). 2000. *Healthy People 2010: Understanding and Improving Health.* 2nd ed. Washington, DC: U.S. Government Printing Office.

DHHS/USDA (U.S. Department of Agriculture). 2004. *Report of the Dietary Guidelines Advisory Committee on the Dietary Guidelines for Americans, 2005. A Report to the Secretary of Health and Human Services and the Secretary of Agriculture.* [Online]. Available: http://www.health.gov/dietaryguidelines/dga2005/report/ [accessed November 28, 2006].

DHHS/USDA. 2005. *Dietary Guidelines for Americans 2005.* Washington, DC: U.S. Government Printing Office. [Online]. Available: http://www.health.gov/dietaryguidelines/dga2005/document/ [accessed November 17, 2006].

Fox MK, Crepinsek MK, Connor P, Battaglia M. 2001. School Nutrition Dietary Assessment Study-II (SNDA-II): *Summary of Findings.* Alexandria, VA: Food and Nutrition Service, USDA.

French SA, Story M, Fulkerson JA, Gerlach AF. 2003. Food environment in secondary schools: À la carte, vending machines, and food policies and practices. *Am J Public Health* 93(7):1161–1167.

GAO (U.S. Government Accountability Office). 2005. *School Meal Programs: Competitive Foods Are Widely Available and Generate Substantial Revenues for Schools.* GAO-05-563. Washington, DC: GAO. [Online]. Available: http://www.gao.gov/new.items/d05563.pdf [accessed October 6, 2005].

Gerald DE, Hussar WJ. 2003. *Projections of Educational Statistics to 2013.* NCES 2004-013. Washington, DC: National Center for Education Statistics, U.S. Department of Education.

Gleason P, Suitor C. 2001. *Children's Diets in the Mid-1990s: Dietary Intake and Its Relationship with School Meal Participation.* Report No. CN-01-CD1. Alexandria, VA: Office of Analysis, Nutrition and Evaluation, Food and Nutrition Service, USDA.

Harnack L, Snyder P, Story M, Holliday R, Lytle L, Neumark-Sztainer D. 2000. Availability of a la carte food items in junior and senior high schools: A needs assessment. *J Am Diet Assoc* 100(6):701–703.

IOM (Institute of Medicine). 1997. *Dietary Reference Intakes for Calcium, Phosphorus, Magnesium, Vitamin D, and Fluoride.* Washington, DC: National Academy Press.

IOM. 1998. *Dietary Reference Intakes for Thiamin, Riboflavin, Niacin, Vitamin B6, Folate, Vitamin B12, Pantothenic Acid, Biotin, and Choline.* Washington, DC: National Academy Press.

IOM. 2000. *Dietary Reference Intakes for Vitamin C, Vitamin E, Selenium, and Carotenoids.* Washington, DC: National Academy Press.

IOM. 2001. *Dietary Reference Intakes for Vitamin A, Vitamin K, Arsenic, Boron, Chromium, Copper, Iodine, Iron, Manganese, Molybdenum, Nickel, Silicon, Vanadium, and Zinc.* Washington, DC: National Academy Press.

IOM. 2002/2005. *Dietary Reference Intakes for Energy, Carbohydrate, Fiber, Fat, Fatty Acids, Cholesterol, Protein, and Amino Acids.* Washington, DC: The National Academies Press.

IOM. 2005a. *Dietary Reference Intakes for Water, Potassium, Sodium, Chloride, and Sulfate.* Washington, DC: The National Academies Press.

IOM. 2005b. *Preventing Childhood Obesity: Health in the Balance.* Washington, DC: The National Academies Press.

IOM. 2006. *Food Marketing to Children and Youth: Threat or Opportunity?* Washington, DC: The National Academies Press.

IOM. 2007. *Progress in Preventing Childhood Obesity: How Do We Measure Up?* Washington, DC: The National Academies Press.

Kubik MY, Lytle LA, Hannan PJ, Perry CL, Story M. 2003. The association of the school food environment with dietary behaviors of young adolescents. *Am J Public Health* 93(7):1168–1173.

Kubik MY, Lytle LA, Story M. 2005. Schoolwide food practices are associated with body mass index in middle school students. *Arch Pediatr Adolesc Med* 159(12):1111–1114.

Lear JG, Isaacs SL, Knickman JR. 2006. *School Health Services and Programs.* San Francisco, CA: Jossey-Bass.

Lytle LA, Kubik MY. 2003. Nutritional issues for adolescents. *Best Pract Res Clin Endocrinol Metab* 17(2):177–189.

Parsad B, Lewis L. 2006. *Calories In, Calories Out: Food and Exercise in Public Elementary Schools, 2005.* Washington, DC: National Center for Education Statistics, U.S. Department of Education.

Probart C, McDonnell E, Weirich JE, Hartman T, Bailey-Davis L, Prabhakher V. 2005. Competitive foods available in Pennsylvania public high schools. *J Am Diet Assoc* 105(8):1243–1249.

Templeton SB, Marlette MA, Panemangalore M. 2005. Competitive foods increase the intake of energy and decrease the intake of certain nutrients by adolescents consuming school lunch. *J Am Diet Assoc* 105(2):215–220.

U.S. Census Bureau. 2006. *Statistical Abstract of the United States 2006.* Table 11. Resident Population by Age and Sex: 1980 to 2004. [Online]. Available: http://www.census.gov/compendia/statab/2006edition.html [accessed November 15, 2006].

USDA (U.S. Department of Agriculture). 2005. *My Pyramid.* [Online]. Available: http://www.mypyramid.gov/ [accessed November 17, 2006].

USDA. 2006. *School Meals: Regulations.* USDA, Food and Nutrition Service. [Online]. Available: http://www.fns.usda.gov/cnd/Governance/regulations.htm [accessed January 4, 2007].

Wechsler H, Brener ND, Kuester S, Miller C. 2001. Food service and foods and beverages available at school: Results from the School Health Policies and Programs Study 2000. *J School Health* 71(7): 313–324.

WHO (World Health Organization). 2003. *Joint WHO/FAO Expert Consultation on Diet, Nutrition and the Prevention of Chronic Diseases.* WHO Technical Report Series 916. Geneva: WHO. [Online]. Available: http://www.fao.org/docrep/005/AC911E/AC911E00. HTM [accessed November 20, 2006].

CHAPTER 2

AAP (American Academy of Pediatrics). 2004a. The fourth report on the diagnosis, evaluation, and treatment of high blood pressure in children and adolescents. *Pediatrics* 114(2 Suppl):555–576.

AAP, Committee on Nutrition. 2004b. *Pediatric Nutrition Handbook.* 5th ed. Elk Grove Village, IL: American Academy of Pediatrics.

AAP, Committee on School Health. 2004c. Policy statement. Soft drinks in schools. *Pediatrics* 113(1):152–154.

Abbott PJ. 1986. Caffeine: A toxicological overview. *Med J Aust* 145(10):518–521.

ADA (American Diabetes Association). 2003. Economic costs of diabetes in the U.S. in 2002. *Diabetes Care* 26(3):917–932.

ADA (American Dietetic Association). 2004. Position of the American Dietetic Association: Use of nutritive and nonnutritive sweeteners. *J Am Diet Assoc* 104(2):255–275.

Affenito SG, Thompson DR, Barton BA, Franko DL, Daniels SR, Obarzanek E, Schreiber GB, Striegel-Moore RH. 2005. Breakfast consumption by African-American and white adolescent girls correlates positively with calcium and fiber intake and negatively with body mass index. *J Am Diet Assoc* 105(6):938–945.

Alderman MH. 2002. Salt, blood pressure and health: A cautionary tale. *Int J Epidemiol* 31:311–315.

Allan JR, Wilson CG. 1971. Influence of acclimatization on sweat sodium concentration. *J Appl Physiol* 30(5):708–712.

Allsopp AJ, Sutherland R, Wood P, Wootton SA. 1998. The effect of sodium balance on sweat sodium secretion and plasma aldosterone concentration. *Eur J Applied Physiol* 78:516–521.

APA (American Psychiatric Association). 2000. *Diagnostic and Statistical Manual of Mental Disorders: DSM-IV.* 4th text revision ed. Washington, DC: APA Press.

Bachman CM, Baranowski T, Nicklas TA. 2006. Is there an association between sweetened beverages and adiposity? *Nutr Rev* 64(4):153–174.

Baer RA. 1987. Effects of caffeine on classroom behavior, sustained attention, and a memory task in preschool children. *J Appl Behav Anal* 20(3):225–234.

Bankel M, Eriksson UC, Robertson A, Kohler B. 2006. Caries and associated factors in a group of Swedish children 2–3 years of age. *Swed Dent J* 30(4):137–146.

Bao W, Threefoot SA, Srinivasan SR, Berenson GS. 1995. Essential hypertension predicted by tracking of elevated blood pressure from childhood to adulthood: The Bogalusa Heart Study. *Am J Hypertens* 8:657–665.

Barton BA, Eldridge AL, Thompson D, Affenito SG, Striegel-Moore RH, Franko DL, Albertson AM, Crockett SJ. 2005. The relationship of breakfast and cereal consumption to nutrient intake and body mass index: The National Heart, Lung, and Blood Institute Growth and Health Study. *J Am Diet Assoc* 105(9):1383–1389.

Beard JL. 2000. Iron requirements in adolescent females. J Nutr 130(2S Suppl):440S–442S.

Beltran-Aguilar ED, Barker LK, Canto MT, Dye BA, Gooch BF, Griffin SO, Hyman J, Jaramillo F, Kingman A, Nowjack-Raymer R, Selwitz RH, Wu T. 2005. Surveillance for dental caries, dental sealants, tooth retention, edentulism, and enamel fluorosis—United States, 1988–1994 and 1999–2002. MMWR Surveill Summ 54(3):1–43.

Benton D. 2004. Role of parents in the determination of the food preferences of children and the development of obesity. Int J Obes Relat Metab Disord 28(7):858–869.

Berenson GS, Srinivasan SR, Bao W, Newman WP, Tracy RE, Wattigney WA. 1998. Association between multiple cardiovascular risk factors and atherosclerosis in children and young adults. N Engl J Med 338(23):1650–1656.

Bernstein GA, Carroll ME, Thuras PD, Cosgrove KP, Roth ME. 2002. Caffeine dependence in teenagers. Drug Alcohol Depend 66(1):1–6.

Birch LL. 1998. Development of food acceptance patterns in the first years of life. Proc Nutr Soc 57(4):617–624.

Birch LL. 1999. Development of food preferences. Annu Rev Nutr 19:41–62.

Birch LL, Fisher JO. 1998. Development of eating behaviors among children and adolescents. Pediatrics 101(3 Pt 2):539–549.

Bjelakovic G, Nikolova D, Simonetti RG, Gluud C. 2004. Antioxidant supplements for prevention of gastrointestinal cancers: A systematic review and meta-analysis. Lancet 364(9441):1219–1228.

Blackburn GL, Kanders BS, Lavin PT, Keller SD, Whatley J. 1997. The effect of aspartame as part of a multidisciplinary weight-control program on short- and long-term control of body weight. Am J Clin Nutr 65(2):409–418.

Blum JW, Jacobsen DJ, Donnelly JE. 2005. Beverage consumption patterns in elementary school aged children across a two-year period. J Am Coll Nutr 24(2):93–98.

Bowman SA. 1999. Diets of individuals based on energy intakes from added sugars. Fam Econ Nutr Rev 12(2):31–38.

Bowman SA. 2002. Beverage choices of young females: Changes and impact on nutrient intakes. J Am Diet Assoc 102(9):1234–1239.

Bowman SA, Gortmaker SL, Ebbeling CB, Pereira MA, Ludwig DS. 2004. Effects of fast-food consumption on energy intake and diet quality among children in a national household survey. Pediatrics 113(1 Pt 1):112–118.

Briefel RR, Johnson CL. 2004. Secular trends in dietary intake in the United States. Annu Rev Nutr 24:401–431.

Butchko HH, Stargel WW. 2001. Aspartame: Scientific evaluation in the postmarketing period. Regul Toxicol Pharmacol 34(3):221–233.

Butte NF. 2006. Energy requirements of infants and children. Nestle Nutr Workshop Ser Pediatr Program 58:19–32.

CDC (Centers for Disease Control and Prevention). 1998. Recommendations to prevent and control iron deficiency in the United States. MMWR Morb Mortal Wkly Rep 47(RR-3):1–29.

CDC. 1999. Achievements in public health, 1900–1999: Safer and healthier foods. MMWR Morb Mortal Wkly Rep 48(40):905–913.

CDC. 2000. CDC Growth Charts: United States 2000. [Online]. Available: www.cdc.gov/growthcharts [accessed May 30, 2006].

CDC. 2002. Iron deficiency—United States, 1999–2000. MMWR Morb Mortal Wkly Rep 51(40):897–899.

CDC/DHHS (U.S. Department of Health and Human Services). 2006. Preventing Chronic Diseases: Investing Wisely in Health. Preventing Dental Caries. Atlanta, GA: CDC.

Cleveland LE, Moshfegh AJ, Albertson AM, Goldman JD. 2000. Dietary intake of whole grains. J Am Coll Nutr 19(3):331S–338S.

Cook S, Weitzman M, Auinger P, Nguyen M, Dietz WH. 2003. Prevalence of a metabolic syndrome phenotype in adolescents: Findings from the Third National Health and Nutrition Examination Survey, 1988–1994. *Arch Pediatr Adolesc Med* 157(8):821–827.

Cross AT, Babicz D, Cushman LF. 1994. Snacking patterns among 1,800 adults and children. *J Am Diet Assoc* 94(12):1398–1403.

Curatolo PW, Robertson D. 1983. The health consequences of caffeine. *Ann Intern Med* 98(5 Pt 1):641–653.

Daniels SR. 2006. The consequences of childhood overweight and obesity. *Future Child* 16(1):47–67.

Dekkers JC, Snieder H, Van Den Oord EJ, Treiber FA. 2002. Moderators of blood pressure development from childhood to adulthood: A 10-year longitudinal study. *J Pediatr* 141(6):770–779.

Deshmukh-Taskar P, Nicklas TA, Morales M, Yang SJ, Zakeri I, Berenson GS. 2006. *Tracking of overweight status from childhood to young adulthood: The Bogalusa Heart Study. Eur J Clin Nutr* 60(1):48–57.

Devaney BL, Gordon AR, Burghardt JA. 1995. Dietary intakes of students. *Am J Clin Nutr* 61(1 Suppl):205S–212S.

Devaney B, Kim M, Carriquiry A, Camano-Garcia G. 2005. *Assessing the Nutrient Intakes of Vulnerable Subgroups.* Electronic report from the Economic Research Service, U.S. Department of Agriculture. [Online]. Available: http://www.ers.usda.gov/Publications/ CCR11/ [accessed February 27, 2007].

Dews PB, O'Brien CP, Bergman J. 2002. Caffeine: Behavioral effects of withdrawal and related issues. *Food Chem Toxicol* 40(9):1257–1261.

DHHS (U.S. Department of Health and Human Services). 2000. *Healthy People 2010: Understanding and Improving Health.* 2nd ed. Washington, DC: U.S. Government Printing Office.

DHHS. 2004a. *Bone Health and Osteoporosis: A Report of the Surgeon General.* Rockville, MD: Office of the Surgeon General, DHHS.

DHHS. 2004b. *Child Health USA 2004.* Rockville, MD: U.S. DHHS.

DHHS/USDA (DHHS/U.S. Department of Agriculture). 2004. *Report of the Dietary Guidelines Advisory Committee on the Dietary Guidelines for Americans, 2005. A Report to the Secretary of Health and Human Services and the Secretary of Agriculture.* [Online]. Available: http://www.health.gov/dietaryguidelines/dga2005/report/ [accessed November 28, 2006].

DHHS/USDA. 2005. *Dietary Guidelines for Americans 2005.* Washington, DC: U.S. Government Printing Office. [Online]. Available: http://www.health.gov/dietaryguidelines/ dga2005/document/ [accessed November 17, 2006].

Dietz WH. 2006. Sugar-sweetened beverages, milk intake, and obesity in children and adolescents. *J Pediatr* 148(2):152–154.

Dixit A, Vaney N, Tandon OP. 2006. Evaluation of cognitive brain functions in caffeine users: A P3 evoked potential study. *Indian J Physiol Pharmacol* 50(2):175–180.

Dorfman LJ, Jarvik ME. 1970. Comparative stimulant and diuretic actions of caffeine and theobromine in man. *Clin Pharmacol Ther* 11(6):869–872.

Drewnowski A. 1997. Taste preferences and food intake. *Annu Rev Nutr* 17:237–253.

Dye BA, Shenkin JD, Ogden CL, Marshall TA, Levy SM, Kanellis MJ. 2004. The relationship between healthful eating practices and dental caries in children aged 2–5 years in the United States, 1988–1994. *J Am Dent Assoc* 135(1):55–66.

Eaton DK, Kann L, Kinchen S, Ross J, Hawkins J, Harris WA, Lowry R, McManus T, Chyen D, Shanklin S, Lim C, Grunbaum JA, Wechsler H. 2006. Youth risk behavior surveillance—United States, 2005. *MMWR Surveill Summ* 55(5):1–108.

Ebbeling CB, Feldman HA, Osganian SK, Chomitz VR, Ellenbogen SJ, Ludwig DS. 2006. Effects of decreasing sugar-sweetened beverage consumption on body weight in adolescents: A randomized, controlled pilot study. *Pediatrics* 117(3):673–680.

EFSA (European Food Safety Authority). 2006. Opinion of the scientific panel AFC related to a new long-term carcinogenicity study on aspartame. *The EFSA Journal* 356:1–44. [Online]. Available: http://www.efsa.europa.eu/en/science/afc/afc_opinions/1471.html [accessed January 3, 2007].

Emans SJ. 2000. Eating disorders in adolescent girls. *Pediatr Int* 42(1):1–7.

Enns CW, Mickle SJ, Goldman JD. 2002. Trends in food and nutrient intakes by children in the United States. *Fam Econ Nutr Rev* 14(2):56–68.

Enns CW, Mickle SJ, Goldman JD. 2003. Trends in food and nutrient intakes by adolescents in the United States. *Fam Econ Nutr Rev* 15(2):15–27.

Erikson GC, Hager LB, Houseworth C, Dungan J, Petros T, Beckwith BE. 1985. The effects of caffeine on memory for word lists. *Physiol Behav* 35(1):47–51.

FAO/WHO/UNU (Food and Agriculture Organization of the United Nations/World Health Organization/United Nations University). 2004. *Human Energy Requirements.* Rome, Italy: WHO. [Online]. Available: http://www.fao.org/docrep/007/y5686e/y5686e00. HTM [accessed March 16, 2007].

FDA (U.S. Food and Drug Administration). 2006a. *Artificial sweeteners: No calories . . . .sweet!* FDA Consumer Magazine 40(4). [Online]. Available: http://www.fda.gov/fdac/406_toc. html [accessed January 27, 2007].

FDA. 2006b. *Guidance for Industry and Staff. Whole Grain Label Statements. Draft Guidance.* College Park, MD: Center for Food Safety and Applied Nutrition, FDA. [Online]. Available: http://www.cfsan.fda.gov/~dms/flgragui.html [accessed January 12, 2006].

FIFCFS (Federal Interagency Forum on Child and Family Statistics). 2005. *America's Children: Key National Indicators of Well-Being, 2005.* Washington, DC: U.S. Government Printing Office.

Fisher JO, Birch LL. 1999. Restricting access to palatable foods affects children's behavioral response, food selection, and intake. *Am J Clin Nutr* 69(6):1264–1272.

Fisher JO, Mitchell DC, Smiciklas-Wright H, Birch LL. 2002. Parental influences on young girls' fruit and vegetable, micronutrient, and fat intakes. *J Am Diet Assoc* 102(1):58–64.

Fisher JO, Mitchell DC, Smiciklas-Wright H, Mannino ML, Birch LL. 2004. Meeting calcium recommendations during middle childhood reflects mother-daughter beverage choices and predicts bone mineral status. *Am J Clin Nutr* 79(4):698–706.

Foltin RW, Fischman MW, Moran TH, Rolls BJ, Kelly TH. 1990. Caloric compensation for lunches varying in fat and carbohydrate content by humans in a residential laboratory. *Am J Clin Nutr* 52(6):969–980.

Fox MK, Cole N. 2004. *Nutrition and Health Characteristics of Low-Income Populations. Vol. III, School-Age Children.* Report No. E-FAN-04-014-3. Washington, DC: Economic Research Service, U.S. Department of Agriculture.

FRAC (Food Research and Action Center). 2006. *State of the States: 2006. A Profile of Food and Nutrition Programs Across the Nation.* Washington, DC: FRAC.

Franco V, Oparil S. 2006. Salt sensitivity, a determinant of blood pressure, cardiovascular disease and survival. *J Am Coll Nutr* 25 (3 Suppl):247S–255S.

Frary CD, Johnson RK, Wang MQ. 2004. Children and adolescents' choices of foods and beverages high in added sugars are associated with intakes of key nutrients and food groups. *J Adolesc Health* 34(1):56–63.

Frary CD, Johnson RK, Wang MQ. 2005. Food sources and intakes of caffeine in the diets of persons in the United States. *J Am Diet Assoc* 105(1):110–113.

Freedman DS, Dietz WH, Srinivasan SR, Berenson GS. 1999. The relation of overweight to cardiovascular risk factors among children and adolescents: The Bogalusa Heart Study. *Pediatrics* 103(6):1175–1182.

French SA, Story M, Neumark-Sztainer D, Fulkerson JA, Hannan P. 2001. Fast food restaurant use among adolescents: Associations with nutrient intake, food choices and behavioral and psychosocial variables. *Int J Obes* 25(12):1823–1833.

French SA, Lin BH, Guthrie JF. 2003. National trends in soft drink consumption among children and adolescents age 6 to 17 years: Prevalence, amounts, and sources, 1977/1978 to 1994/1998. *J Am Diet Assoc* 103(10):1326–1331.

Geleijnse JM, Grobbee DE, Hofman A. 1990. Sodium and potassium intake and blood pressure change in childhood. *Br Med J* 300:899–902.

Geleijnse JM, Hofman A, Witteman JCM, Hazebroek AAJM, Valenburg HA, Grobbee DE. 1997. Long-term effects of neonatal sodium restriction on blood pressure. *Hypertension* 29:913–917.

Gidding SS, Dennison BA, Birch LL, Daniels SR, Gilman MW, Lichtenstein AH, Rattay KT, Steinberger J, Stettler N, Van Horn L. 2005. Dietary recommendations for children and adolescents: A guide for practitioners. Consensus Statement from the American Heart Association. *Circulation* 112(13):2061–2075.

Gidding SS, Dennison BA, Birch LL, Daniels SR, Gilman MW, Lichtenstein AH, Rattay KT, Steinberger J, Stettler N, Van Horn L. 2006. Dietary recommendations for children and adolescents: A guide for practitioners. *Pediatrics* 117(2):544–559.

Gillman MW, Cook NR, Rosner B, Evans DA, Keough ME, Taylor JO, Hennekens CH. 1993. Identifying children at high risk for the development of essential hypertension. *J Pediatr* 122:837–846.

Gillman MW, Rifas-Shiman S, Frazier L, Rockett H, Camargo C, Field A, Berkey C, Colditz G. 2000. Family dinner and diet quality among older children and adolescents. *Archives of Family Medicine* 9(3):235–240.

Gleason P, Suitor C. 2001a. *Children's Diets in the Mid-1990s: Dietary Intake and Its Relationship with School Meal Participation.* Report No. CN-01-CD1. Alexandria, VA: Office of Analysis, Nutrition and Evaluation, Food and Nutrition Service, U.S. Department of Agriculture.

Gleason P, Suitor C. 2001b. *Food for Thought: Children's Diets in the 1990s.* Princeton, NJ: Mathematica Policy Research, Inc.

Goran MI. 1998. Measurement issues related to studies of childhood obesity: Assessment of body composition, body fat distribution, physical activity, and food intake. *Pediatrics* 101(3 Pt 2):505–518.

Grandjean AC, Reimers KJ, Bannick KE, Haven MC. 2000. The effect of caffeinated, non-caffeinated, caloric and non-caloric beverages on hydration. *J Am Coll Nutr* 19(5):591–600.

Grantham-McGregor S, Ani C. 2001. A review of studies on the effect of iron deficiency on cognitive development in children. *J Nutr* 131(2S-2):649S–668S.

Green PJ, Suls J. 1996. The effects of caffeine on ambulatory blood pressure, heart rate, and mood in coffee drinkers. *J Behav Med* 19(2):111–128.

Greer FR, Krebs NF. 2006. Optimizing bone health and calcium intakes of infants, children, and adolescents. *Pediatrics* 117(2):578–585.

Griffiths RR, Chausmer AL. 2000. Caffeine as a model drug of dependence: Recent developments in understanding caffeine withdrawal, the caffeine dependence syndrome, and caffeine negative reinforcement. *Nihon Shinkei Seishin Yakurigaku Zasshi* 20(5):223–231.

Griffiths RR, Woodson PP. 1988. Caffeine physical dependence: A review of human and laboratory animal studies. *Psychopharmacology* (Berl) 94(4):437–451.

Grundy SM. 1999. The optimal ratio of fat-to-carbohydrate in the diet. *Annu Rev Nutr* 19:325–341.

Guthrie JF, Morton JF. 2000. Food sources of added sweeteners in the diets of Americans. *J Am Diet Assoc* 100(1):43–51.

Halterman JS, Kaczorowski JM, Aligne CA, Auinger P, Szilagyi PG. 2001. Iron deficiency and cognitive achievement among school-aged children and adolescents in the United States. *Pediatrics* 107(6):1381–1386.

Hanson NI, Neumark-Sztainer D, Eisenberg ME, Story M, Wall M. 2005. Associations between parental report of the home food environment and adolescent intakes of fruits, vegetables, and dairy foods. *Public Health Nutr* 8(1):77–85.

Harnack L, Stang J, Story M. 1999. Soft drink consumption among U.S. children and adolescents: Nutritional consequences. *J Am Diet Assoc* 99(4):436–441.

Harnack L, Walters SA, Jacobs DR. 2003. Dietary intake and food sources of whole grains among U.S. children and adolescents: Data from the 1994–1996 Continuing Survey of Food Intakes by Individuals. *J Am Diet Assoc* 103(8):1015–1019.

Heaney RP. 2000. Calcium, dairy products and osteoporosis. *J Am Coll Nutr* 19(2): 83S–99S.

Heaney RP, Abrams S, Dawson-Hughes B, Looker A, Marcus R, Matkovic V, Weaver C. 2000. Peak bone mass. *Osteoporos Int* 11(12):985–1009.

Heatherley SV, Hancock KM, Rogers PJ. 2006. Psychostimulant and other effects of caffeine in 9- to 11-year-old children. *J Child Psychol Psychiatry* 47(2):135–142.

Higdon JV, Frei B. 2006. Coffee and health: A review of recent human research. *Crit Rev Food Sci Nutr* 46(2):101–123.

Huang T, Howarth NC, Lin BH, Roberts SB, McCrory MA. 2004. Energy intake and meal portions: Associations with BMI percentile in U.S. children. *Obes Res* 12(11):1875–1885.

Hughes JR, Hale KL. 1998. Behavioral effects of caffeine and other methylxanthines on children. *Exp Clin Psychopharmacol* 6(1):87–95.

IOM (Institute of Medicine). 1993. *Nutritional Needs in Hot Environments: Applications for Military Personnel in Field Operations.* Washington, DC: National Academy Press.

IOM. 1996. *Nutritional Needs in Cold and in High-Altitude Environments: Applications for Military Personnel in Field Operations.* Washington, DC: National Academy Press.

IOM. 1997. *Dietary Reference Intakes for Calcium, Phosphorus, Magnesium, Vitamin D, and Fluoride.* Washington, DC: National Academy Press.

IOM. 1998. *Dietary Reference Intakes for Thiamin, Riboflavin, Niacin, Vitamin B6, Folate, Vitamin B12, Pantothenic Acid, Biotin, and Choline.* Washington, DC: National Academy Press.

IOM. 2000. *Dietary Reference Intakes for Vitamin C, Vitamin E, Selenium, and Carotenoids.* Washington, DC: National Academy Press.

IOM. 2001. *Dietary Reference Intakes for Vitamin A, Vitamin K, Arsenic, Boron, Chromium, Copper, Iodine, Iron, Manganese, Molybdenum, Nickel, Silicon, Vanadium, and Zinc.* Washington, DC: National Academy Press.

IOM. 2002/2005. *Dietary Reference Intakes for Energy, Carbohydrate, Fiber, Fat, Fatty Acids, Cholesterol, Protein and Amino Acids.* Washington, DC: The National Academies Press.

IOM. 2005a. *Dietary Reference Intakes for Water, Potassium, Sodium, Chloride, and Sulfate.* Washington, DC: The National Academies Press.

IOM. 2005b. *Preventing Childhood Obesity: Health in the Balance.* Washington, DC: The National Academies Press.

IOM. 2007. *Progress in Preventing Childhood Obesity: How Do We Measure Up?* Washington, DC: The National Academies Press.

Jago R, Harrell JS, Mcmurray RG, Edelstein S, El Ghormli L, Bassin S. 2006. Prevalence of abnormal lipid and blood pressure values among an ethnically diverse population of eighth-grade adolescents and screening implications. *Pediatrics* 117(6):2065–2073.

Jahns L, Siega-Riz AM, Popkin BM. 2001. The increasing prevalence of snacking among U.S. children from 1977 to 1996. *J Pediatr* 138(4):493–498.

James J, Thomas P, Cavan D, Kerr D. 2004. Preventing childhood obesity by reducing consumption of carbonated drinks: Cluster randomised controlled trial. *Br Med J* 328(7450): 1237–1241.

James JE. 1997. Is habitual caffeine use a preventable cardiovascular risk factor? *Lancet* 349(9047):279–281.

Jeffery E. 2005. Component interactions for efficacy of functional foods. *J Nutr* 135(5): 1223–1225.

Johnson RK. 2000. What are people really eating and why does it matter? *Nutrition Today* 35(2):40–46.

Johnson RK, Frary C, Wang MQ. 2002. The nutritional consequences of flavored-milk consumption by school-aged children and adolescents in the United States. *J Am Diet Assoc* 102(6):853–856.

Kant AK. 2003. Reported consumption of low-nutrient-density foods by American children and adolescents: Nutritional and health correlates, NHANES III, 1988 to 1994. *Arch Pediatr Adolesc Med* 157(8):789–796.

Kenemans JL, Lorist MM. 1995. Caffeine and selective visual processing. *Pharmacol Biochem Behav* 52(3):461–471.

Lader MH. 1999. Caffeine withdrawal. In: Gupta BS, Gupta U, eds. *Caffeine and Behavior: Current Views and Research Trends*. Boca Raton, FL: CRC Press. Pp. 151–178.

Leonard TK, Watson RR, Mohs ME. 1987. The effects of caffeine on various body systems: A review. *J Am Diet Assoc* 87(8):1048–1053.

Leviton A. 1992. Behavioral correlates of caffeine consumption by children. *Clin Pediatr (Phila)* 31(12):742–750.

Lim U, Subar AF, Mouw T, Hartge P, Morton LM, Stolzenberg-Solomon R, Campbell D, Hollenbeck AR, Schatzkin A. 2006. Consumption of aspartame-containing beverages and incidence of hematopoietic and brain malignancies. *Cancer Epidemiol Biomarkers Prev* 15(9):1654–1659.

Lin BH, Morrison RM. 2002. Higher fruit consumption linked with lower body mass index. *FoodReview* 25(3):28–32.

Lin BH, Guthrie J, Frazao E. 2001. American children's diets not making the grade. *FoodReview* 24(2):8–17.

Lingstrom P, Holm AK, Mejare I, Twetman S, Soder B, Norlund A, Axelsson S, Lagerlof F, Nordenram G, Petersson LG, Dahlgren H, Kallestal C. 2003. Dietary factors in the prevention of dental caries: A systematic review. *Acta Odontol Scand* 61(6):331–340.

Liu RH. 2004. Potential synergy of phytochemicals in cancer prevention: Mechanism of action. *J Nutr* 134(12 Suppl):3479S–3485S.

Loke WH. 1988. Effects of caffeine on mood and memory. *Physiol Behav* 44(3):367–372.

Ludwig DS, Peterson KE, Gortmaker SL. 2001. Relation between consumption of sugar-sweetened drinks and childhood obesity: A prospective, observational analysis. *Lancet* 357(9255):505–508.

Lytle LA, Seifert S, Greenstein J, McGovern P. 2000. How do children's eating patterns and food choices change over time? Results from a cohort study. *Am J Health Promot* 14(4):222–228.

Malik VS, Schulze MB, Hu FB. 2006. Intake of sugar-sweetened beverages and weight gain: A systematic review. *Am J Clin Nutr* 84(2):274–288.

Mannino ML, Lee Y, Mitchell DC, Smiciklas-Wright H, Birch LL. 2004. The quality of girls' diets declines and tracks across middle childhood. *Int J Behav Nutr Phys Act* 1(1):5.

Manson MM. 2003. Cancer prevention—the potential for diet to modulate molecular signalling. *Trends Mol Med* 9(1):11–18.

Marshall TA, Eichenberger-Gilmore JM, Broffitt B, Stumbo PJ, Levy SM. 2005. Diet quality in young children is influenced by beverage consumption. *J Am Coll Nutr* 24(1):65–75.

Marshall TA, Eichenberger-Gilmore JM, Larson MA, Warren JJ, Levy SM. 2007. Comparison of the intakes of sugars by young children with and without dental caries experience. *J Am Dent Assoc* 138(1):39–46.

Martin RM, McCarthy A, Smith GD, Davies DP, Ben-Shlomo Y. 2003. Infant nutrition and blood pressure in early adulthood: The Barry Caerphilly Growth Study. *Am J Clin Nutr* 77(6):1489–1497.

Maurer J, Taren DL, Teixeira PJ, Thomson CA, Lohman TG, Going SB, Houtkooper LB. 2006. The psychosocial and behavioral characteristics related to energy misreporting. *Nutr Rev* 64(2 Pt 1):53–66.

McCusker RR, Goldberger BA, Cone EJ. 2006. Caffeine content of energy drinks, carbonated sodas, and other beverages. *J Anal Toxicol* 30(2):112–114.

Melgar-Quinonez HR, Kaiser LL. 2004. Relationship of child-feeding practices to overweight in low-income Mexican-American preschool-aged children. *J Am Diet Assoc* 104(7):1110–1119.

Mennella JA, Pepino MY, Reed DR. 2005. Genetic and environmental determinants of bitter perception and sweet preferences. *Pediatrics* 115(2):e216–e222.

Mennella JA, Kennedy JM, Beauchamp GK. 2006. Vegetable acceptance by infants: Effects of formula flavors. *Early Hum Dev* 82(7):463–468.

Miech RA, Kumanyika SK, Stettler N, Link BG, Phelan JC, Chang VW. 2006. Trends in the association of poverty with overweight among U.S. adolescents, 1971–2004. *J Am Med Assoc* 295(20):2385–2393.

Miller ER, 3rd, Pastor-Barriuso R, Dalal D, Riemersma RA, Appel LJ, Guallar E. 2005. Meta-analysis: High-dosage vitamin E supplementation may increase all-cause mortality. *Ann Intern Med* 142(1):37–46.

Moshfegh A, Goldman J, Cleveland L. 2005. *What We Eat in America, NHANES 2001–2002: Usual Nutrient Intakes from Food Compared to Dietary Reference Intakes*. Agriculture Research Service, U.S. Department of Agriculture. [Online]. Available: http://www.ars.usda.gov/Services/docs.htm?docid=9098 [accessed Dec 6, 2005].

Moynihan P, Petersen PE. 2004. Diet, nutrition and the prevention of dental diseases. *Public Health Nutr* 7(1A):201–226.

Mrdjenovic G, Levitsky DA. 2003. Nutritional and energetic consequences of sweetened drink consumption in 6- to 13-year-old children. *J Pediatr* 142(6):604–610.

Munoz KA, Krebs-Smith SM, Ballard-Barbash R, Cleveland LE. 1997. Food intakes of U.S. children and adolescents compared with recommendations. *Pediatrics* 100(3):323–329.

Munoz KA, Krebs-Smith SM, Ballard-Barbash R, Cleveland LE. 1998. Errors in food intake article. *Pediatrics* 101(5):952–953.

Muntner P, He J, Cutler JA, Wildman RP, Whelton PK. 2004. Trends in blood pressure among children and adolescents. *J Am Med Assoc* 291(17):2107–2113.

Myers MG. 2004. Effect of caffeine on blood pressure beyond the laboratory. *Hypertension* 43(4):724–725.

Narayan KMV, Boyle JP, Thompson TJ, Sorensen SW, Williamson DF. 2003. Lifetime risk for diabetes mellitus in the United States. *J Am Med Assoc* 290(14):1884–1890.

Neuhouser ML, Patterson RE, Thornquist MD, Omenn GS, King IB, Goodman GE. 2003. Fruits and vegetables are associated with lower lung cancer risk only in the placebo arm of the beta-carotene and retinol efficacy trial (CARET). *Cancer Epidemiol Biomarkers Prev* 12(4):350–358.

Neumark-Sztainer D, Story M, Resnick MD, Blum RW. 1996. Correlates of inadequate fruit and vegetable consumption among adolescents. *Prev Med* 25(5):497–505.

Neumark-Sztainer D, Story M, Perry C, Casey MA. 1999. Factors influencing food choices of adolescents: Findings from focus-group discussions with adolescents. *J Am Diet Assoc* 99(8):929–937.

Neumark-Sztainer D, Hannan PJ, Story M, Croll J, Perry C. 2003. Family meal patterns: Associations with sociodemographic characteristics and improved dietary intake among adolescents. *J Am Diet Assoc* 103(3):317–322.

Neumark-Sztainer D, Hannan PJ, Story M, Perry CL. 2004. Weight-control behaviors among adolescent girls and boys: Implications for dietary intake. *J Am Diet Assoc* 104(6):913–920.

Neumark-Sztainer D, Wall M, Guo J, Story M, Haines J, Eisenberg M. 2006. Obesity, disordered eating, and eating disorders in a longitudinal study of adolescents: How do dieters fare 5 years later? *J Am Diet Assoc* 106(4):559–568.

Nicklas TA, Bao W, Webber LS, Berenson GS. 1993. Breakfast consumption affects adequacy of total daily intake in children. *J Am Diet Assoc* 93(8):886–891.

Nicklas TA, Morales M, Linares A, Yang SJ, Baranowski T, De Moor C, Berenson G. 2004. Children's meal patterns have changed over a 21-year period: The Bogalusa Heart Study. *J Am Diet Assoc* 104(5):753–761.

Nielsen SJ, Popkin BM. 2004. Changes in beverage intake between 1977 and 2001. *Am J Prev Med* 27(3):205–210.

Nielsen SJ, Siega-Riz AM, Popkin BM. 2002. Trends in food locations and sources among adolescents and young adults. *Prev Med* 35(2):107–113.

NIH (National Institutes of Health). 2006. National Institutes of Health State-of-the-science conference statement: Multivitamin/mineral supplements and chronic disease prevention. *Ann Intern Med* 145(5):364–371.

Nussberger J, Mooser V, Maridor G, Juillerat L, Waeber B, Brunner HR. 1990. Caffeine-induced diuresis and atrial natriuretic peptides. *J Cardiovasc Pharmacol* 15(5):685–691.

Oberstar JV, Bernstein GA, Thuras PD. 2002. Caffeine use and dependence in adolescents: One-year follow-up. *J Child Adolesc Psychopharmacol* 12(2):127–135.

O'Brien CP. 1995. Drug addiction and drug abuse. In: Hardman JG, Limbird LE, eds. *Goodman and Gilman's The Pharmacological Basis of Therapeutics*. 9th ed. New York: Macmillan. Pp. 557–577.

O'Dea JA. 2003. Why do kids eat healthful food? Perceived benefits of and barriers to healthful eating and physical activity among children and adolescents. *J Am Diet Assoc* 103(4):497–501.

Ogden CL, Flegal KM, Carroll MD, Johnson CL. 2002. Prevalence and trends in overweight among U.S. children and adolescents, 1999–2000. *J Am Med Assoc* 288(14): 1728–1732.

Ogden CL, Carroll MD, Curtin LR, McDowell MA, Tabak CJ, Flegal KM. 2006. Prevalence of overweight and obesity in the United States, 1999–2004. *J Am Med Assoc* 295(13):1549–1555.

Passmore AP, Kondowe GB, Johnston GD. 1987. Renal and cardiovascular effects of caffeine: A dose-response study. *Clin Sci* 72(6):749–756.

Pereira MA. 2006. The possible role of sugar-sweetened beverages in obesity etiology: A review of the evidence. *Int J Obes* 30(Suppl 3):S28–S36.

Pham DQ, Plakogiannis R. 2005. Vitamin E supplementation in cardiovascular disease and cancer prevention: Part 1. *Ann Pharmacother* 39(11):1870–1878.

Pollitt E, Mathews R. 1998. Breakfast and cognition: An integrative summary. *Am J Clin Nutr* 67(4):804S–813S.

Popkin BM, Armstrong LE, Bray GM, Caballero B, Frei B, Willett WC. 2006. A new proposed guidance system for beverage consumption in the United States. *Am J Clin Nutr* 83(3):529–542.

Porikos KP, Booth G, Van Itallie TB. 1977. Effect of covert nutritive dilution on the spontaneous food intake of obese individuals: A pilot study. *Am J Clin Nutr* 30(10):1638–1644.

Porikos KP, Hesser MF, Van Itallie TB. 1982. Caloric regulation in normal-weight men maintained on a palatable diet of conventional foods. *Physiol Behav* 29(2):293–300.

Prentice AM. 2001. Obesity and its potential mechanistic basis. *Br Med Bull* 60(1):51–67.

Putnam J, Allshouse J, Kantor LS. 2002. U.S. per capita food supply trends: More calories, refined carbohydrates, and fats. *FoodReview* 25(3):2–15.

Raben A, Vasilaras TH, Moller AC, Astrup A. 2002. Sucrose compared with artificial sweeteners: Different effects on ad libitum food intake and body weight after 10 wk of supplementation in overweight subjects. *Am J Clin Nutr* 76(4):721–729.

Raitakari OT, Juonala M, Viikari JS. 2005. Obesity in childhood and vascular changes in adulthood: Insights into the Cardiovascular Risk in Young Finns Study. *Int J Obes* 29(S2):S101–S104.

Rajeshwari R, Wang S-J, Nicklas TA, Berensen GS. 2005. Secular trends in children's sweetened-beverage consumption (1973–1994): The Bogalusa Heart Study. *J Am Diet Assoc* 105(2):208–214.

Rampersaud GC, Pereira MA, Girard BL, Adams J, Metzl JD. 2005. Breakfast habits, nutritional status, body weight, and academic performance in children and adolescents. *J Am Diet Assoc* 105(5):743–760.

Rapoport JL, Elkins R, Neims A, Zahn T, Berg CJ. 1981. Behavioral and autonomic effects of caffeine in normal boys. *Dev Pharmacol Ther* 3(2):74–82.

Rapoport JL, Berg CJ, Ismond DR, Zahn TP, Neims A. 1984. Behavioral effects of caffeine in children. *Arch Gen Psychiatry* 41(11):1073–1079.

Reeves RR, Struve FA, Patrick G, Bullen JA. 1995. Topographic quantitative EEG measures of alpha and theta power changes during caffeine withdrawal: Preliminary findings from normal subjects. *Clin Electroencephalogr* 26(3):154–162.

Renwick AG. 1990. Acceptable daily intake and the regulation of intense sweeteners. *Food Addit Contam* 7(4):463–475.

Ritchie LD, Ivey SL, Woodward-Lopez G, Crawford PB. 2003. Alarming trends in pediatric overweight in the United States. *Soz Preventivmed* 48(3):168–177.

Rodriguez BL, Fujimoto WY, Mayer-Davis EJ, Imperatore G, Williams DE, Bell RA, Wadwa RP, Palla SL, Liu LL, Kershnar A, Daniels SR, Linder B. 2006. Prevalence of cardiovascular disease risk factors in U.S. children and adolescents with diabetes: The SEARCH for Diabetes in Youth Study. *Diabetes Care* 29(8):1891–1896.

Rogers PJ, Blundell JE. 1989. Separating the actions of sweetness and calories: Effects of saccharin and carbohydrates on hunger and food intake in human subjects. *Physiol Behav* 45(6):1093–1099.

Rolls BJ, Ello-Martin JA, Tohill BC. 2004. What can intervention studies tell us about the relationship between fruit and vegetable consumption and weight management? *Nutr Rev* 62(1):1–17.

Rolls BJ, Roe LS, Meengs JS. 2006. Larger portion sizes lead to a sustained increase in energy intake over 2 days. *J Am Diet Assoc* 106(4):543–549.

Rome ES, Ammerman S, Rosen DS, Keller RJ, Lock J, Mammel KA, O'Toole J, Rees JM, Sanders MJ, Sawyer SM, Schneider M, Sigel E, Silber TJ. 2003. Children and adolescents with eating disorders: The state of the art. *Pediatrics* 111(1):e98–e108.

Siega-Riz AM, Popkin BM, Carson T. 1998. Trends in breakfast consumption for children in the United States from 1965–1991. *Am J Clin Nutr* 67(4):748S–756S.

Slavin JL, Jacobs D, Marquart L, Wiemer K. 2001. The role of whole grains in disease prevention. *J Am Diet Assoc* 101(7):780–785.

Soffritti M. 2006. Acesulfame potassium: Soffritti responds. *Environ Health Perspect* 114(9): A516–A517.

Soffritti M, Belpoggi F, Esposti DD, Lambertini L. 2005. Aspartame induces lymphomas and leukaemias in rats. *Eur J Oncol* 10(2):107–116.

Sorof JM, Lai D, Turner J, Poffenbarger T, Portman RJ. 2004. Overweight, ethnicity, and the prevalence of hypertension in school-aged children. *Pediatrics* 113(3):475–482.

Storey ML, Forshee RA, Anderson PA. 2004. Associations of adequate intake of calcium with diet, beverage consumption, and demographic characteristics among children and adolescents. *J Am Coll Nutr* 23(1):18–33.

Story M, Neumark-Sztainer D, Sherwood N, Stang J, Murray D. 1998. Dieting status and its relationship to eating and physical activity behaviors in a representative sample of U.S. adolescents. *J Am Diet Assoc* 98(10):1127–1135.

Story M, Holt K, Sofka D. 2002a. *Bright Futures in Practice: Nutrition*. 2nd ed. Arlington, VA: National Center for Education in Maternal and Child Health. [Online]. Available: http://www.brightfutures.org/nutrition/pdf/index.html [accessed November 20, 2006].

Story M, Lytle LA, Birnbaum AS, Perry CL. 2002b. Peer-led, school-based nutrition education for young adolescents: Feasibility and process evaluation of the TEENS study. *J Sch Health* 72(3):121–127.

Striegel-Moore RH, Thompson D, Affenito SG, Franko DL, Obarzanek E, Barton BA, Schreiber GB, Daniels SR, Schmidt M, Crawford PB. 2006. Correlates of beverage intake in adolescent girls: The National Heart, Lung, and Blood Institute Growth and Health Study. *J Pediatr* 148(2):183–187.

Sturm R. 2005. Childhood obesity—What we can learn from existing data on societal trends, Part 2. *Prev Chronic Dis* 2(2):A20.

Subar AF, Krebs-Smith SM, Cook A, Kahle LL. 1998. Dietary sources of nutrients among U.S. children, 1989–1991. *Pediatrics* 102(4 Pt 1):913–923.

Terry WS, Phifer B. 1986. Caffeine and memory performance on the AVLT. *J Clin Psychol* 42(6):860–863.

Thompson OM, Ballew C, Resnicow K, Must A, Bandini LG, Cyr H, Dietz WH. 2004. Food purchased away from home as a predictor of change in BMI z-score among girls. *Int J Obes* 28(2):282–289.

Thorpe LE, List DG, Marx T, May L, Helgerson SD, Frieden TR. 2004. Childhood obesity in New York City elementary school students. *Am J Public Health* 94(9):1496–1500.

Tordoff MG, Alleva AM. 1990. Effect of drinking soda sweetened with aspartame or high-fructose corn syrup on food intake and body weight. *Am J Clin Nutr* 51(6):963–969.

Touger-Decker R, Mobley CC. 2003. Position of the American Dietetic Association: Oral health and nutrition. *J Am Diet Assoc* 103(5):615–625.

Touger-Decker R, van Loveren C. 2003. Sugars and dental caries. *Am J Clin Nutr* 78(4):881S–892S.

Troiano RP, Briefel RR, Carroll MD, Bialostosky K. 2000. Energy and fat intakes of children and adolescents in the United States: Data from the National Health and Nutrition Examination Surveys. *Am J Clin Nutr* 72(5 Suppl):1343S–1353S.

Umemura T, Ueda K, Nishioka K, Hidaka T, Takemoto H, Nakamura S, Jitsuiki D, Soga J, Goto C, Chayama K, Yoshizumi M, Higashi Y. 2006. Effects of acute administration of caffeine on vascular function. *Am J Cardiol* 98(11):1538–1541.

USDA/ARS (U.S. Department of Agriculture/Agricultural Research Service). 2006. *USDA Nutrient Database for Standard Reference, Release 19*. [Online]. Available: http://www.ars.usda.gov/nutrientdata [accessed January 26, 2007].

USDA/ERS (USDA/Economic Research Service). 2006. Food Security in the United States: Measuring Household Food Security. [Online]. Available: http://www.ers.usda.gov/Briefing/FoodSecurity/measurement.htm [accessed March 26, 2007].

USPSTF (U.S. Preventive Services Task Force). 2003. Routine vitamin supplementation to prevent cancer and cardiovascular disease: Recommendations and rationale. *Ann Intern Med* 139(1):51–55.

Van Lenthe FJ, Kemper HCG, Twisk JWR. 1994. Tracking of blood pressure in children and youth. *Am J Hum Biol* 6:389–399.

Vartanian LR, Schwartz MB, Brownell KD. 2007. Effects of soft drink consumption on nutrition and health: A systematic review and meta-analysis. *Am J Public Health* 97(4):667–675.

Videon TM, Manning CK. 2003. Influences on adolescent eating patterns: The importance of family meals. *J Adolesc Health* 32(5):365–373.

Wang Y, Zhang Q. 2006. Are American children and adolescents of low socioeconomic status at increased risk of obesity? Changes in the association between overweight and family income between 1971 and 2002. *Am J Clin Nutr* 84(4):707–716.

Wang YC, Gortmaker SL, Sobal AM, Kuntz KM. 2006. Estimating the energy gap among U.S. children: A counterfactual approach. *Pediatrics* 118(6):1721–1733.

Weaver CM, Heaney RP. 2006. Calcium. In: Shils ME, Shike M, Ross AC, Caballero B, Cousins RJ, eds. *Modern Nutrition in Health and Disease*. 10th ed. Philadelphia, PA: Lippincott, Williams, and Wilkins.

Weaver CM, Peacock M, Johnston CC. 1999. Adolescent nutrition in the prevention of post-menopausal osteoporosis. *J Clin Endocrinol Metab* 84(6):1839–1843.

Weihrauch MR, Diehl V. 2004. Artificial sweeteners—do they bear a carcinogenic risk? *Ann Oncol* 15(10):1460–1465.

Weiss R, Dziura J, Burgert TS, Tamborlane WV, Taksali SE, Yeckel CW, Allen K, Lopes M, Savoye M, Morrison J, Sherwin RS, Caprio S. 2004. Obesity and the metabolic syndrome in children and adolescents. *N Engl J Med* 350(23):2362–2374.

Welsh JA, Cogswell ME, Rogers S, Rockett H, Mei Z, Grummer-Strawn LM. 2005. Overweight among low-income preschool children associated with the consumption of sweet drinks: Missouri, 1999–2002. *Pediatrics* 115(2):e223–e229.

Whiting SJ, Healey A, Psiuk S, Mirwald R, Kowalski K, Bailey DA. 2001. Relationship between carbonated and other low nutrient dense beverages and bone mineral content of adolescents. *Nutr Res* 21(8):1101–1115.

WHO (World Health Organization). 2003. *Joint WHO/FAO Expert Consultation on Diet, Nutrition and the Prevention of Chronic Diseases*. WHO Technical Report Series 916. Geneva, Switzerland: WHO. [Online]. Available: http://www.fao.org/docrep/005/AC911E/AC911E00.HTM [accessed November 20, 2006].

Williams CL, Hayman LL, Daniels SR, Robinson TN, Steinberger J, Paridon S, Bazzarre T. 2002. Cardiovascular health in childhood: A statement for health professionals from the Committee on Atherosclerosis, Hypertension, and Obesity in the Young (AHOY) of the Council on Cardiovascular Disease in the Young, American Heart Association. *Circulation* 106(1):143–160.

Winkelmayer WC, Stampfer MJ, Willett WC, Curhan GC. 2005. Habitual caffeine intake and the risk of hypertension in women. *J Am Med Assoc* 294(18):2330–2335.

Yen ST, Lin B-H. 2002. Beverage consumption among U.S. children and adolescents: Full information and quasi maximum-likelihood estimation of a censored system. *Eur Rev Agric Econ* 29(1):85–103.

Young LR, Nestle M. 2002. The contribution of expanding portion sizes to the U.S. obesity epidemic. *Am J Public Health* 92(2):246–249.

Zero DT. 2004. Sugars—the arch criminal? *Caries Res* 38(3):277–285.

Zizza C, Siega-Riz AM, Popkin BM. 2001. Significant increase in young adults' snacking between 1977–1978 and 1994–1996 represents a cause for concern! *Prev Med* 32(4):303–310.

CHAPTER 3

ASFSA (American School Food Service Association). 2002. *À la Carte and Vending Research Program: Summary Report*. Alexandria, VA: ASFSA.

Baranowski T, Baranowski J, Cullen KW, Marsh T, Islam N, Zakeri I, Honess-Morreale L, deMoor C. 2003a. Squire's Quest! Dietary outcome evaluation of a multimedia game. *Am J Prev Med* 24(1):52–61.

Baranowski T, Cullen KW, Nicklas T, Thompson DI, Baranowski J. 2003b. Are current health behavioral change models helpful in guiding prevention of weight gain efforts? *Obes Res* 11(Suppl):23S–43S.

Briggs M, Safaii S, Beall DL. 2003. Position of the American Dietetic Association, Society for Nutrition Education, and American School Food Service Association—Nutrition services: An essential component of comprehensive school health programs. *J Am Diet Assoc* 103(4):505–514.

Burghardt J, Gordon A, Chapman N, Gleason P, Fraker T. 1993. *The School Nutrition Dietary Assessment Study (SNDA-I): Final Report*. Alexandria, VA: Food and Nutrition Service, U.S. Department of Agriculture.

CDC (Centers for Disease Control and Prevention). 2006. Secondary school health education related to nutrition and physical activity—selected sites, United States, 2004. *MMWR Morb Mortal Wkly Rep* 55(30)821–824.

Contento I, Balch GI, Bronner M. 1995. The effectiveness of nutrition education and implications for nutrition education policy, programs and research: A review of research. *J Nutr Educ* 27(6):277–422.

Cullen KW, Zakeri I. 2004. Fruits, vegetables, milk, and sweetened beverage consumption and access to a la carte/snack bar meals at school. *Am J Public Health* 94(3):463–467.

DASH (Centers for Disease Control and Prevention's Division of Adolescent and School Health). 2006. *Healthy School, Healthy Youth! 2006*. [Online]. Available: http://www.cdc.gov/HealthyYouth/ [accessed May 24, 2006].

DHHS (U.S. Department of Health and Human Services). 2000. *Healthy People 2010: Understanding and Improving Health*. 2nd ed. Washington, DC: U.S. Government Printing Office.

DHHS/USDA (U.S. Department of Agriculture). 2005. *Dietary Guidelines for Americans 2005*. Washington, DC: U.S. Government Printing Office. [Online]. Available: http://www.health.gov/dietaryguidelines/dga2005/document/ [accessed November 17, 2006].

Doak CM, Visscher TL, Renders CM, Seidell JC. 2006. The prevention of overweight and obesity in children and adolescents: A review of interventions and programmes. *Obes Rev* 7(1):111–136.

Eaton DK, Kann L, Kinchen S, Ross J, Hawkins J, Harris WA, Lowry R, McManus T, Chyen D, Shanklin S, Lim C, Grunbaum JA, Wechsler H. 2006. Youth risk behavior surveillance—United States, 2005. *MMWR Surveil Summ* 55(5):1–108.

Flynn MA, McNeil DA, Maloff B, Mutasingwa D, Wu M, Ford C, Tough SC. 2006. Reducing obesity and related chronic disease risk in children and youth: A synthesis of evidence with "best practice" recommendations. *Obes Rev* 7(Suppl 1):7–66.

French SA, Story M, Fulkerson JA, Gerlach AF. 2003. Food environment in secondary schools: A la carte, vending machines, and food policies and practices. *Am J Public Health* 93(7):1161–1167.

GAO (U.S. Government Accountability Office). 2000. *Public Education: Commercial Activities in Schools*. GAO/HEHS-00-156. Washington, DC: GAO. [Online]. Available: http://www.gao.gov/archive/2000/he00156.pdf [accessed December 6, 2006].

GAO. 2003. *School Lunch Program: Efforts Needed to Improve Nutrition and Encourage Healthy Eating.* GAO-03-506. Washington, DC: GAO. [Online]. Available: http://www. gao.gov/new.items/d03506.pdf [accessed December 6, 2006].

GAO. 2004. *School Meal Programs: Competitive Foods are Available in Many Schools; Actions Taken to Restrict Them Differ by State and Locality.* GAO-04-673. Washington, DC: GAO.

GAO. 2005. *School Meal Programs: Competitive Foods Are Widely Available and Generate Substantial Revenues for Schools.* GAO-05-563. Washington, DC: GAO. [Online]. Available: http://www.gao.gov/new.items/d05563.pdf [accessed October 6, 2005].

Graham H, Zidenberg-Cherr S. 2005. California teachers perceive school gardens as an effective nutritional tool to promote healthful eating habits. *J Am Diet Assoc* 105(11):1797–1800.

Hoelscher DM, Kelder SH, Murray N, Cribb PW, Conroy J, Parcel GS. 2001. Dissemination and adoption of the Child and Adolescent Trial for Cardiovascular Health (CATCH): A case study in Texas. *J Public Health Manag Pract* 7(2):90–100.

IOM (Institute of Medicine). 2002/2005. *Dietary Reference Intakes for Energy, Carbohydrate, Fiber, Fat, Fatty Acids, Cholesterol, Protein, and Amino Acids.* Washington, DC: The National Academies Press.

IOM. 2006. *Food Marketing to Children and Youth: Threat or Opportunity?* Washington, DC: The National Academies Press.

Kann L, Brener ND, Allensworth DD. 2001. Health education: Results from the School Health Policies and Programs Study 2000. *J Sch Health* 71(7):266–278.

Kubik MY, Lytle LA, Hannan PJ, Perry CL, Story M. 2003. The association of the school food environment with dietary behaviors of young adolescents. *Am J Public Health* 93(7):1168–1173.

Liquori T, Koch PD, Contento IR, Castle J. 1998. The Cookshop Program: Outcome evaluation of nutrition education program linking lunchroom food experiences with classroom cooking experiences. *J Nutr Educ* 30(5):302–313.

Luepker RV, Perry CL, McKinlay SM, Nader PR, Parcel GS, Stone EJ, Webber LS, Elder JP, Feldman HA, Johnson CC. 1996. Outcomes of a field trial to improve children's dietary patterns and physical activity. The Child and Adolescent Trial for Cardiovascular Health. CATCH collaborative group. *J Am Med Assoc* 275(10):768–776.

Lytle L, Achterberg C. 1995. Changing the diet of America's children: What works and why? *J Nutr Educ* 27(5):250–260.

Lytle L, Gerlach S, Weinstein AB. 2001. Conducting nutrition education research in junior high schools: Approaches and challenges. *J Nutr Educ* 33(1):49–54.

Lytle LA, Murray DM, Perry CL, Story M, Birnbaum AS, Kubik MY, Varnell S. 2004. School-based approaches to affect adolescents' diets: Results from the TEENS study. *Health Educ Behav* 31(2):270–287.

Lytle LA, Kubik MY, Perry C, Story M, Birnbaum AS, Murray DM. 2006. Influencing healthful food choices in school and home environments: Results from the TEENS study. *Prev Med* 43(1):8–13.

Maras E. 2004. State of the vending industry report. *Automatic Merchandiser.* [Online]. Available: http://www.amonline.com/reports/index.jsp [accessed December 9, 2006].

NASPE/AHA (National Association for Sport and Physical Education/American Heart Association). 2006. *2006 Shape of the Nation Report: Status of Physical Education in the USA.* Reston, VA: NASPE.

Nestle M. 2000. Soft drink "pouring rights": Marketing empty calories to children. *Public Health Rep* 115(4):308–319.

Neumark-Sztainer D, Story M, Perry C, Casey MA. 1999. Factors influencing food choices of adolescents: Findings from focus-group discussions with adolescents. *J Am Diet Assoc* 99(8):929–937.

O'Dea JA. 2003. Why do kids eat healthful food? Perceived benefits of and barriers to healthful eating and physical activity among children and adolescents. *J Am Diet Assoc* 103(4):497–501.

O'Neil CE, Nicklas TA. 2002. Gimme 5: An innovative, school-based nutrition intervention for high school students. *J Am Diet Assoc* 102(3 Suppl):S93–S96.

Orrell-Valente JK, Hill LG, Brechwald WA, Dodge KA, Pettit GS, Bates JE. 2007. "Just three more bites": An observational analysis of parents' socialization of children's eating at mealtime. *Appetite* 48(1):37–45.

Palmer E, Cantor J, Dowrick P, Kunkel D, Linn S, Wilcox B. 2004. Psychological implications of commercialism in schools. In: *Report of the APA Task Force on Advertising and Children*. Washington, DC: American Psychological Association. [Online]. Available: http://www.apa.org/releases/childrenads.html [accessed January 24, 2007].

Perry CL, Bishop DB, Taylor GL, Davis M, Story M, Gray C, Bishop SC, Mays RA, Lytle LA, Harnack L. 2004. A randomized school trial of environmental strategies to encourage fruit and vegetable consumption among children. *Health Educ Behav* 31(1):65–76.

Ritchie LD, Welk G, Styne D, Gerstein DE, Crawford PB. 2005. Family environment and pediatric overweight: What is a parent to do? *J Am Diet Assoc* 105 (5 Suppl 1):S70–S79.

Story M, French S. 2004. Food advertising and marketing directed at children and adolescents in the U.S. *Int J Behav Nutr Phys Act* 1(1):3.

Story M, Kaphingst KM, French S. 2006. The role of schools in obesity prevention. *The Future of Children* 16(1):109–142.

Templeton SB, Marlette MA, Panemangalore M. 2005. Competitive foods increase the intake of energy and decrease the intake of certain nutrients by adolescents consuming school lunch. *J Am Diet Assoc* 105(2):215–220.

USDA/CDC (U.S. Department of Agriculture/Centers for Disease Control and Prevention). 2005. *Making it Happen! School Nutrition Success Stories*. Alexandria, VA: Food and Nutrition Service, USDA.

Wechsler H, Brener ND, Kuester S, Miller C. 2001. Food service and foods and beverages available at school: Results from the School Health Policies and Programs Study 2000. *J School Health* 71(7):313–324.

Whitaker RC, Wright JA, Koepsell TD, Finch AJ, Psaty BM. 1994. Randomized intervention to increase children's selection of low-fat foods in school lunches. *J Pediatr* 125(4):535–540.

Woodward-Lopez G, Vargas A, Kim S, Proctor C, Hiort-Lorenzen Diemoz L, Crawford P. 2005. *LEAF Cross-Site Evaluation: Fiscal Impact Report*. Center for Weight and Health, University of California, Berkeley. [Online]. Available: http://www.cnr.berkeley.edu/cwh/activities/LEAF.shtml [accessed December 8, 2006].

WVDE (West Virginia Department of Education). 2004. Standards for School Nutrition (4321.1). Title 126. Legislative Rule. Board of Education. Series 86. [Online]. Available: http://wvde.state.wv.us/policies/p4321.1.html [accessed March 26, 2007].

CHAPTER 4

ABA (American Beverage Association). 2005. *Beverage Industry Announces New School Vending Policy: Plan Calls For Lower-Calorie and/or Nutritious Beverages in Schools and New Limits on Soft Drinks*. [Online]. Available: http://www.ameribev.org/news-detail/index.aspx?nid=53 [accessed December 13, 2006].

ABA. 2006. *School Beverage Guidelines.* Washington, DC: ABA.

Alliance for a Healthier Generation. 2006. *Competitive Food Guidelines.* [Online]. Available: http://www.healthiergeneration.org/engine/renderpage.asp?pid=s042 [accessed December 13, 2006].

APHA (American Public Health Association). 2003. *Support for WIC and Child Nutrition Programs.* Washington, DC: APHA. [Online]. Available: http://www.apha.org/legislative/policy/policysearch/index.cfm?fuseaction=view&id=1257 [accessed December 12, 2006].

Burros M, Warner M. 2006. *Bottlers agree to a school ban on sweet drinks.* The New York Times, May 4, A1.

CSPI (Center for Science in the Public Interest). 2006. *School Foods Report Card. A State-by-State Evaluation of Policies for Foods and Beverages Sold Through Vending Machines, School Stores, À La Carte, and Other Venues Outside of School Meals.* [Online]. Available: http://cspinet.org/new/pdf/school_foods_report_card.pdf [accessed December 6, 2006].

DHHS/USDA (U.S. Department of Health and Human Services/U.S. Department of Agriculture). 2005. *Dietary Guidelines for Americans 2005.* Washington, DC: U.S. Government Printing Office. [Online]. Available: http://www.health.gov/dietaryguidelines/dga2005/document/ [accessed November 17, 2006].

FRAC (Food Research and Action Center). 2006. *State of the States: 2006. A Profile of Food and Nutrition Programs Across the Nation.* Washington, DC: FRAC.

GAO (U.S. Government Accountability Office). 2004. *School Meal Programs: Competitive Foods are Available in Many Schools; Actions Taken to Restrict Them Differ by State and Locality.* GAO-04-673. Washington, DC: GAO.

GAO. 2005. *School Meal Programs: Competitive Foods Are Widely Available and Generate Substantial Revenues for Schools.* GAO-05-563. Washington, DC: GAO. [Online]. Available: http://www.gao.gov/new.items/d05563.pdf [accessed October 6, 2005].

Garnett S, Eadie R, Miller C. 2006 (April 21). *School Meal Programs: Lessons Learned.* Presentation to the Institute of Medicine, Food and Nutrition Board, Committee on Nutrition Standards in Schools, Washington, DC.

Gleason P, Suitor C. 2001. *Children's Diets in the Mid-1990s: Dietary Intake and Its Relationship with School Meal Participation.* Report No. CN-01-CD1. Alexandria, VA: Office of Analysis, Nutrition and Evaluation, Food and Nutrition Service, U.S. Department of Agriculture.

Greves HM, Rivara FP. 2006. Report card on school snack food policies among the United States' largest school districts in 2004–2005: Room for improvement. *Int J Behav Nutr Phys Act* 3(1). [Online]. Available: http://www.ijbnpa.org/content/3/1/1 [accessed June 12, 2006].

Griffith P, Sackin B, Bierbauer D. 2000 (May 30). *School Meals: Benefits and Challenges. White Paper for the National Nutrition Summit.* Alexandria, VA: American School Food Service Association.

HPTS (Health Policy Tracking Service). 2004. *Nutrition, Obesity, and Physical Education: 2004 Overview.* NETSCAN iPublishing Inc. [Online]. Available: http://www.rwjf.org/files/research/NCSL%202004%20End%20of%20Year%20Report.pdf [accessed April 10, 2007].

HPTS. 2005a (April 4). *School Nutrition and Physical Education Legislation: An Overview of 2005 State Activity.* NETSCAN iPublishing Inc. [Online]. Available: http://www.rwjf.org/files/research/NCSL%20-%20April%202005%20Quarterly%20Report.pdf [accessed April 10, 2007].

HPTS. 2005b (December 31). *State Actions to Promote Nutrition, Increase Physical Activity and Prevent Obesity: A Legislative Overview.* Health Policy Tracking Service, A Thomson West Business. [Online]. Available: http://www.rwjf.org/files/research/RWJFDecReport.pdf [accessed April 10, 2007].

HPTS. 2006 (April 3). *State Actions to Promote Nutrition, Increase Physical Activity and Prevent Obesity: A 2006 First Quarter Legislative Overview.* NetScan's Health Policy Tracking Service, a service of Thomson West. [Online]. Available: http://www.rwjf.org/files/research/NCSL%20FinalApril%202006%20Report.pdf [accessed April 10, 2007].

HPTS. 2007 (February 8). *Nutritional Standards for Competitive Foods Sold in Elementary, Middle, or High School.* Health Policy Tracking Service, a service of Thomson West.

NANA (National Alliance for Nutrition and Activity). 2005. *Update USDA's School Nutrition Standards: Cosponsor the Child Nutrition Promotion and School Lunch Protection Act.* Washington, DC: Center for Science in the Public Interest.

Neumark-Sztainer D, French SA, Hannan PJ, Story M, Fulkerson JA. 2005. School lunch and snacking patterns among high school students: Associations with school food environment and policies. *Int J Behav Nutr Phys Act* 2(1):14.

Samuels and Associates. 2006. *Competitive Foods. Policy Brief.* Oakland, CA: Samuels & Associates. [Online]. Available: http://www.calendow.org/reference/publications/pdf/disparities/Competitive%20Foods%20Brief.pdf [accessed December 12, 2006].

Story M, Kaphingst KM, French S. 2006. The role of schools in obesity prevention. *The Future of Children* 16(1):109–142.

Trust for America's Health. 2006. *F as in Fat: How Obesity Policies are Failing in America.* Washington, DC: Trust for America's Health. [Online]. Available: http://healthyamericans.org/reports/obesity2006/ [accessed December 12, 2006].

USDA (U.S. Department of Agriculture). 2001. *Foods Sold in Competition with the USDA School Meal Programs: A Report to Congress.* [Online]. Available: http://www.fns.usda.gov/cnd/Lunch/CompetitiveFoods/report_congress.htm [accessed December 12, 2006].

USDA/CDC (USDA/Centers for Disease Control and Prevention). 2005. *Making It Happen! School Nutrition Success Stories.* Alexandria, VA: Food and Nutrition Service, USDA.

Wechsler H, Brener ND, Kuester S, Miller C. 2001. Food service and foods and beverages available at school: Results from the School Health Policies and Programs Study 2000. *J School Health* 71(7): 313–324.

CHAPTER 5

AAP (American Academy of Pediatrics), Committee on Nutrition. 2001. The use and misuse of fruit juice in pediatrics. *Pediatrics* 107(5):1210–1213.

Cleveland LE, Moshfegh AJ, Albertson AM, Goldman JD. 2000. Dietary intake of whole grains. *J Am Coll Nutr* 19(3):331S–338S.

DHHS/USDA (U.S. Department of Health and Human Services/U.S. Department of Agriculture). 2004. *Report of the Dietary Guidelines Advisory Committee on the Dietary Guidelines for Americans, 2005. A Report to the Secretary of Health and Human Services and the Secretary of Agriculture.* [Online]. Available: http://www.health.gov/dietaryguidelines/dga2005/report/ [accessed November 28, 2006].

DHHS/USDA. 2005. *Dietary Guidelines for Americans 2005.* Washington, DC: U.S. Government Printing Office. [Online]. Available: http://www.health.gov/dietaryguidelines/dga2005/document/ [accessed November 17, 2006].

GAO (U.S. Government Accountablility Office). 2003. *School Lunch Program: Efforts Needed to Improve Nutrition and Encourage Healthy Eating*. GAO-03-506. Washington, DC: GAO. [Online]. Available: http://www.gao.gov/new.items/d03506.pdf [accessed December 6, 2006].

GAO. 2004. *School Meal Programs: Competitive Foods are Available in Many Schools; Actions Taken to Restrict Them Differ by State and Locality*. GAO-04-673. Washington, DC: GAO.

GAO. 2005. *School Meal Programs: Competitive Foods Are Widely Available and Generate Substantial Revenues for Schools*. GAO-05-563. Washington, DC: GAO. [Online]. Available: http://www.gao.gov/new.items/d05563.pdf [accessed October 6, 2005].

Guenther PM, Dodd KW, Reedy J, Krebs-Smith SM. 2006. Most Americans eat much less than recommended amounts of fruits and vegetables. *J Am Diet Assoc* 106(9):1371–1379.

USDA (U.S. Department of Agriculture). 2005. *USDA National Nutrient Database for Standard Reference Release 18*. [Online]. Available: http://www.nal.usda.gov/fnic/foodcomp/Data/SR18/sr18.html [Accessed November 20, 2006].

WHO (World Health Organization). 2003. *Joint WHO/FAO Expert Consultation on Diet, Nutrition and the Prevention of Chronic Diseases*. WHO Technical Report Series 916. Geneva, Switzerland: WHO. [Online]. Available: http://www.fao.org/docrep/005/AC911E/AC911E00.HTM [accessed November 20, 2006].

Acronyms and Glossary

ORGANIZATIONS, PROGRAMS, STUDIES

AAP	American Academy of Pediatrics
ABA	American Beverage Association
AHA	American Heart Association
AMA	American Medical Association
ASFSA	American School Food Service Association
CACFP	Child and Adult Care Food Program
CDC	Center for Disease Control and Prevention, U.S. Department of Health and Human Services
CFR	Code of Federal Regulations
CFSAN	Center for Food Safety and Applied Nutrition, U.S. Food and Drug Administration
CNP	Child Nutrition Programs, U.S. Department of Agriculture
CSFII	Continuing Survey of Food Intakes by Individuals
CSHP	Coordinated School Health Program
CSPI	Center for Science in the Public Interest
DASH	Division of Adolescent and School Health, Center for Disease Control and Prevention, U.S. Department of Health and Human Services
DGA (or DG)	Dietary Guidelines for Americans
DHHS	Department of Health and Human Services
FAO	Food and Agriculture Organization

FDA	Food and Drug Administration
FNB	Food and Nutrition Board, Institute of Medicine
FNS	Food and Nutrition Service, U.S. Department of Agriculture
GAO	Government Accountability Office
HPTS	Health Policy Tracking Service
IDFA	International Dairy Foods Association
IOM	Institute of Medicine, The National Academies
LEAF	Linking Education, Activity, and Food Evaluation Report
NANA	National Alliance for Nutrition and Activity
NAS	National Academy of Sciences, The National Academies
NASBE	National Association of State Boards of Education
NASPE	National Association for Sport and Physical Education
NCI	National Cancer Institute
NCLB	No Child Left Behind
NDL	Nutrient Data Laboratory, U.S. Department of Agriculture
NDS-R	Nutrient Data System for Research
NFCS	Nationwide Food Consumption Survey
NHANES	National Health and Nutrition Examination Survey
NIH	National Institutes of Health, U.S. Department of Health and Human Services
NSBA	National School Boards Association
NSDA	National Soft Drink Association
NSLP	National School Lunch Program
PCRM	Physicians Committee for Responsible Medicine
RWJ	Robert Wood Johnson Foundation
SBP	School Breakfast Program
SFA	School Food Authority
SHHPS	School Health Policies and Programs
SNA	School Nutrition Association
SNDA-1	School Nutrition Dietary Assessment
SNE	Society for Nutrition Education
SR-17	Standard Reference 17, Nutrient Data Laboratory, U.S. Department of Agriculture
SR-18	Standard Reference 18, Nutrient Data Laboratory, U.S. Department of Agriculture
USDA	U.S. Department of Agriculture
WHO	World Health Organization
WIC	Special Supplemental Nutrition Program for Women, Infants, and Children

TERMS

AI	Adequate intake
BMI	Body mass index
c	Cup or cups
CVD	Cardiovascular disease
d	Day or days
DRI	Dietary Reference Intakes
EAR	Estimated Average Requirement
EER	Estimated Energy Requirement
fl oz	Fluid ounce or fluid ounces
FMNV	Foods of Minimal Nutritional Value
FY	Fiscal year
g	Gram or grams
hr	Hour or hours
kcal	Kilocalorie or kilocalories
kg	Kilogram or kilograms
L	Liter or liters
lb	Pound or pounds
LD	Licensed Dietitian
LDL	Low-density lipoprotein or lipoproteins
mg	Milligram or milligrams
mL	Milliliter or milliliters
mo	Month or months
n	Sample size
N/A	Not applicable
ND	Not determined
oz	Ounce or ounces
oz equiv	Ounce-equivalent
PA	Physical activity
PAL	Physical activity level
qt	Quart or quarts
RD	Registered Dietitian
RDA	Recommended Dietary Allowances
SFA	School Food Authority
T2D	Type 2 Diabetes
tsp	Teaspoon or teaspoons
yr	year

GLOSSARY

Alkaloid compounds—Naturally occurring nitrogenous compound, usually of plant origin. Insoluble in water but soluble in organic solvents and can precipitate proteins.

Aspartame—A low calorie nonnutritive sweetener made of aspartic acid and phenylalanine. It should not be consumed by individuals with phenylketonuria, and is unsuitable for cooking because its flavor is changed when heated.

Atherosclerosis—A form of arteriosclerosis in which atheromas (a mass or plaque of degenerated thickened arterial intima) containing cholesterol, lipid material, and lipophages are formed within the intima and inner media of large and medium-sized arteries.

Beta-carotene—A yellow-orange pigment found in fruits and vegetables; it is the most common precursor of vitamin A. The daily human requirement for vitamin A can be met by dietary intake of beta carotene.

Body mass index—BMI is an indirect measure of body fat calculated as the ratio of a person's body weight in kilograms to the square of a person's height in meters.

Caffeine—A plant-derived alkaloid compound (methylxanthine) that has central nervous system stimulating activity. The primary food and beverage sources are coffee, tea, kola nuts, and chocolate.

California LEAF Study—A pilot study on the effects of competitive food and beverage restriction implementation in California school districts conducted by the Center for Weight and Health at the University of California at Berkeley.

Calorie—A kilocalorie is defined as the amount of heat required to change the temperature of one gram of water from 14.5 degrees Celsius to 15.5 degrees Celsius. In this report, calorie is used synonymously with kilocalorie as a unit of measure for energy obtained from food and beverages.

Child Nutrition Programs (CNP)—U.S. Department of Agriculture. Includes the National School Lunch Program (NSLP), School Breakfast Program (SBP), Child and Adult Care Food Program (CACFP) School Food Service Program (SFSP), and Special Milk Program (SMP).

Cholesterol—A monatomic alcohol found in animal fats and oils, bile, blood, brain tissue, milk, egg yolk, myelin sheaths of nerve fibers, liver, kidneys, and adrenal glands.

Competitive Foods—Foods and beverages offered at schools other than meals and snacks served through the federally reimbursed school lunch, breakfast, and after-school snack programs. Competitive food and beverage items may be sold or offered through à la carte lines, snack bars, student stores, vending machines, or school activities such as special fund-raisers, achievement rewards, classroom parties, school celebrations, classroom snacks, and school meetings, but do not include brown bag lunches.

Cyclamate—A salt of cyclamic acid that is used as a nonnutritive sweetener. It is about 30 times as sweet as sugar.

Dental caries—A destructive process causing decalcification of the tooth enamel and leading to continued destruction of enamel and dentin, and cavitation of the tooth.

Dietary Guidelines for Americans—A federal summary of the latest dietary guidance for the public, based on current scientific evidence and medical knowledge, issued by the U.S. Department of Health and Human Services and U.S. Department of Agriculture, and revised every 5 years.

Dietary Reference Intakes—A set of four, distinct nutrient-based reference values that replace the former Recommended Dietary Allowances in the United States. They include Estimated Average Requirements, Recommended Dietary Allowances, Adequate Intakes, and Tolerable Upper Level Intakes.

Diuresis—The secretion and passage of large amounts of urine. Diuresis occurs as a complication of metabolic disorders such as diabetes mellitus, diabetes insipidus, and hypercalcemia, among others.

Epinephrine—A hormone secreted by the adrenal medulla, and released predominant in response to hypoglycemia. It is a potent stimulator of the sympathetic nervous system, being a powerful vasopressor, increasing blood pressure, and stimulating the heart muscle.

Federally Reimbursable School Nutrition Programs—The National School Lunch and Breakfast Programs, as well as summer and after-school programs.

Foods of minimal nutritional value—Foods prohibited by federal regulation for sale in school food service areas during meal periods.

Healthy weight—In children and youth, a level of body fat where comorbidities are not observed. In adults, a BMI between 18.5 and 24.9 kg/m^2.

Hydrogenated oils—Oils in which molecular hydrogen has been added to double bonds in the unsaturated fatty acids of the glycerides. Oils are changed to solid fats.

Hypercholesterolemia—An excess of cholesterol in the blood.

Hypertension—Persistently high arterial blood pressure.

Methylxanthine—A group of naturally occurring agents present in caffeine, theophylline, and theobromine. They act on the central nervous system, stimulate the myocardium, relax smooth muscle, and promote diuresis.

Monosodium glutamate (MSG)—Chemical used to enhance flavor in foods, can cause headaches, a burning sensation, facial pressure, and chest pain when consumed in large quantities.

Nonnutritive sweetener—Nonnutritive sweeteners include aspartame, sucralose, acesulfame-K, neotame, sugar alcohols, and saccharin. These sweeteners provide a sweet taste without providing additional calories (or an insignificant amount of calories, as is the case for aspartame and sugar alcohols).

Norepinephrine—Secreted by neurons, acts as a transmitter substance of the peripheral sympathetic nerve endings and probably of certain synapses in the central nervous system.

Obesity—In this report, obesity in children and adolescents refers to the age- and sex-specific body mass index (BMI) that is equal to or greater than the 95th percentile of the BMI charts of the Centers for Disease Control and Prevention (CDC). "At risk for obesity" in children and adolescents is defined as a BMI for age and sex that is between the 85th and 95th percentiles of the CDC BMI curves. In most children, a BMI level at or above the 95th percentile indicates elevated body fat and reflects the presence or risk of related chronic disease.

Osteoporosis—Bone disorder characterized by abnormal porosity as a result of diminution in the absolute amount of bone.

Phenylalanine—An essential amino acid; it is one of the two linked amino acids in the sugar substitute Aspartame. The genetically determined inability to dispose of excess phenylalanine is known as phenylketonuria or PKU.

Phenylketonuria (PKU)—A congenital, autosomal recessive disease marked by failure to metabolize the amino acid phenylalanine to tyrosine. It results in severe neurological deficits in infancy if it is unrecognized or left untreated.

Phytochemical—Any of the hundreds of natural chemicals present in plants. Many have nutritional value; others are protective (e.g., antioxidants) or cause cell damage (e.g., free radicals).

Saccharin—a sweet, white, powdered, synthetic product derived from coal tar, 300 to 500 times sweeter than sugar, used as a nonnutritive sweetener.

Sodium benzoate—A white, odorless, granular or crystalline powder, used as an antifungal agent.

Sodium bicarbonate—Used as a gastric and systemic antacid.

Sodium phosphate—A chemical that is used as a cathartic.

Stroke—A condition with sudden onset due to acute vascular lesions of the brain.

Theobromine—A white powder obtained from Theobroma cacao, the plant from which chocolate is obtained. It dilates blood vessels in the heart and peripherally. It is used as a mild stimulant and as a diuretic.

Theophylline—An alkaloid caffeine-related substance found in tea or produced synthetically, used as a smooth muscle relaxant, myocardial stimulant, and diuretic.

APPENDIX
B

Energy Requirements

Estimated Energy Requirements for Boys and Girls

In this sample, median physical activity levels (low active PAL) ranged from 1.47 to 1.54 in 5- to 10-year-old children, 1.53 to 1.79 (low active to active PAL) in 11- to 13- year-old children, and 1.63 to 1.89 (active PAL) in 14- to 18-year-olds. Based on this information, appropriate discretionary energy provided as snacks for elementary school children would range between 124 and 169 calories; for middle school children, between 163 and 236 calories, and for high school students, between 210 and 294 calories.

TABLE B-1 Estimated Energy Requirement (EER) for Boys 3 Through 18 Years of Age

Age (y)	Reference Weight (kg)	Reference Height (m)	Total Energy Expenditure (kcal/d)			
			Sedentary PAL	Low Active PAL	Active PAL	Very Active PAL
3	14.3	0.95	1,142	1,304	1,465	1,663
4	16.2	1.02	1,195	1,370	1,546	1,763
5	18.4	1.09	1,255	1,446	1,638	1,874
6	20.7	1.15	1,308	1,515	1,722	1,977
7	23.1	1.22	1,373	1,597	1,820	2,095
8	25.6	1.28	1,433	1,672	1,911	2,205
9	28.6	1.34	1,505	1,762	2,018	2,334
10	31.9	1.39	1,576	1,850	2,124	2,461
11	35.9	1.44	1,666	1,960	2,254	2,615
12	40.5	1.49	1,773	2,088	2,403	2,792
13	45.6	1.56	1,910	2,251	2,593	3,013
14	51	1.64	2,065	2,434	2,804	3,258
15	56.3	1.7	2,198	2,593	2,988	3,474
16	60.9	1.74	2,295	2,711	3,127	3,638
17	64.6	1.75	2,341	2,771	3,201	3,729
18	67.2	1.76	2,358	2,798	3,238	3,779

EER (kcal/d)				Discretionary Energy (kcal/d)			
Sedentary PAL	Low Active PAL	Active PAL	Very Active PAL	Sedentary PAL	Low Active PAL	Active PAL	Very Active PAL
1,162	1,324	1,485	1,683	105	119	134	151
1,215	1,390	1,566	1,783	109	125	141	160
1,275	1,466	1,658	1,894	115	132	149	170
1,328	1,535	1,742	1,997	120	138	157	180
1,393	1,617	1,840	2,115	125	146	166	190
1,453	1,692	1,931	2,225	131	152	174	200
1,530	1,787	2,043	2,359	138	161	184	212
1,601	1,875	2,149	2,486	144	169	193	224
1,691	1,985	2,279	2,640	152	179	205	238
1,798	2,113	2,428	2,817	162	190	219	254
1,935	2,276	2,618	3,038	174	205	236	273
2,090	2,459	2,829	3,283	188	221	255	295
2,223	2,618	3,013	3,499	200	236	271	315
2,320	2,736	3,152	3,663	209	246	284	330
2,366	2,796	3,226	3,754	213	252	290	338
2,383	2,823	3,263	3,804	214	254	294	342

TABLE B-2 Estimated Energy Requirement (EER) for Girls 3 Through 18 Years of Age

Age (y)	Reference Weight (kg)	Reference Height (m)	Total Energy Expenditure (kcal/d)			
			Sedentary PAL	Low Active PAL	Active PAL	Very Active PAL
3	13.9	0.94	1,060	1,223	1,375	1,629
4	15.8	1.01	1,113	1,290	1,455	1,730
5	17.9	1.08	1,169	1,359	1,537	1,834
6	20.2	1.15	1,227	1,431	1,622	1,941
7	22.8	1.21	1,278	1,495	1,699	2,038
8	25.6	1.28	1,340	1,573	1,790	2,153
9	29	1.33	1,390	1,635	1,865	2,248
10	32.9	1.38	1,445	1,704	1,947	2,351
11	37.2	1.44	1,513	1,788	2,046	2,475
12	41.6	1.51	1,592	1,884	2,158	2,615
13	45.8	1.57	1,659	1,967	2,256	2,737
14	49.4	1.6	1,693	2,011	2,309	2,806
15	52	1.62	1,706	2,032	2,337	2,845
16	53.9	1.63	1,704	2,034	2,343	2,858
17	55.1	1.63	1,685	2,017	2,328	2,846
18	56.2	1.63	1,665	1,999	2,311	2,833

EER (kcal/d)				Discretionary Energy (kcal/d)			
Sedentary PAL	Low Active PAL	Active PAL	Very Active PAL	Sedentary PAL	Low Active PAL	Active PAL	Very Active PAL
1,080	1,243	1,395	1,649	97	112	126	148
1,133	1,310	1,475	1,750	102	118	133	158
1,189	1,379	1,557	1,854	107	124	140	167
1,247	1,451	1,642	1,961	112	131	148	176
1,298	1,515	1,719	2,058	117	136	155	185
1,360	1,593	1,810	2,173	122	143	163	196
1,415	1,660	1,890	2,273	127	149	170	205
1,470	1,729	1,972	2,376	132	156	177	214
1,538	1,813	2,071	2,500	138	163	186	225
1,617	1,909	2,183	2,640	146	172	196	238
1,684	1,992	2,281	2,762	152	179	205	249
1,718	2,036	2,334	2,831	155	183	210	255
1,731	2,057	2,362	2,870	156	185	213	258
1,729	2,059	2,368	2,883	156	185	213	259
1,710	2,042	2,353	2,871	154	184	212	258
1,690	2,024	2,336	2,858	152	182	210	257

APPENDIX
C

Nutrition Standards for Competitive Foods Sold in Elementary, Middle, or High School Set by States

Table C-1 summarizes nutrition standards for competitive foods sold in schools, by state. Information in the table is based on detailed analyses, conducted by the Health Policy Tracking Service (HPTS), and includes policies that limit the times or types of competitive foods available for sale in vending machines, cafeterias, school stores, and snack bars.

TABLE C-1 Nutrition Standards For Competitive Foods Sold in Elementary, Middle, or High School

		Nutrition standards for competitive foods sold in schools (includes items sold à la carte, in school stores and/or vending machines)			
State	Grade Level	Does the state have nutritional standards for competitive foods?	Max. calories from fat	Max. calories from saturated fat	Max. % of sugar by weight
Alabama	Elementary, Middle, and High Schools	Yes	Less than 10% Daily Value of total fat	Not specified	Not specified

| Additional restrictions | Max. calories from fat, saturated fat, and sugar by weight | Additional restrictions on vending machine | | Notes |
		Restrictions on beverages sold in vending machines	Restrictions on access to vending machines	
Competitive foods sold through the vending machines, cafeteria snack items, and the school stores must follow the Alabama's Action for Healthy Kids standards. Those guidelines are as follows: In 1 to 1.5 oz serving, these snack foods are: • Low or moderate in fat (Less than 10% Daily Value of total fat) • Have less than 30 g of carbohydrate • Have less than 360 mg of sodium • Contain 5% Daily Value (DV) or more (10% is healthiest) of at least one: Vitamin A, Vitamin C, Iron, or Calcium • Contain fiber (5% Daily Value)	Refer to additional restriction column.	No carbonated soft drinks in elementary schools. Middle schools: 70% of selections in vending machines are to be noncarbonated water, fruit juices, milk products, teas and sports drinks; 30% of selections can be carbonated soft drinks. Of those, at least 50% (15% of total) will be low/no calorie soft drinks. High Schools: 50% of selections in vending machines are to be noncarbonated water, fruit juices, milk products, teas and sports drinks; 50% of selections can be carbonated soft drinks. Of those, at least 50% will be low/no calorie soft drinks.	None	Recommendations of Alabama Department of Education Nutrition Subcommittee: Schools should provide a consistent environment that is conducive to healthful eating behaviors during school hours and during after-school child care programs. The vending and snack food items in this recommendation shall be implemented at the beginning of the 2006-07 school year except when a conflict with previously negotiated contracts exists. The changes for the cafeteria meals and à la carte items will need to be implemented in conjunction with the leadership of the State Child Nutrition Program. Each school's strategic plan for Improving the School Nutrition Environment plan should be completed by April 1, 2006 and ready for implementation with the beginning of the 2006-07 school years.

continued

TABLE C-1 Continued

State	Grade Level	Nutrition standards for competitive foods sold in schools (includes items sold à la carte, in school stores and/or vending machines)			
		Does the state have nutritional standards for competitive foods?	Max. calories from fat	Max. calories from saturated fat	Max. % of sugar by weight
Alaska	Elementary, Middle, and High Schools	No	N/A	N/A	N/A
Arizona	Elementary, Middle, and High Schools	Yes	35%	10%	35%
Arkansas	Elementary	No	N/A	N/A	N/A

| Additional restrictions | Additional restrictions on vending machine | | | |
	Max. calories from fat, saturated fat, and sugar by weight	Restrictions on beverages sold in vending machines	Restrictions on access to vending machines	Notes
No	N/A	None	None	None
School administrators are prohibited from signing food and beverage contracts that include the sale of sugared, carbonated beverages and all other foods of minimal nutritional value on elementary, middle and junior high school campuses.	35%, 10%, 35%	No fruit/vegetable drinks containing less than 100% juice for Elementary Schools and less than 50% juice for Middle and Junior High Schools; Whole milk (4% milk fat); flavored or regular Caffeine/Energy drinks; Sports drinks, Electrolyte-Replacement drinks for Elementary Schools only; Carbonated beverages.	N/A	The Arizona Nutrition Standards, released in January 2006, go into great detail and cannot be fully summarized in a chart. The standards may be found at http://www.ade. state.az.us/ health-safety/cnp/ HB2544/Arizo-naNutritionStandards.pdf.
Prohibits access to in-school vending machines offering food and beverages. Students will not be served, have access to, or be awarded with competitive foods or FMNVs. Only food items that are part of the school's meal will be sold in the cafeteria. School food service departments may not sell or give extra serving of desserts, french fries, or ice cream.	N/A	Prohibits in-school access to vending machines offering foods and beverages.	Prohibits access to in-school vending machines offering foods and beverages.	None

continued

TABLE C-1 Continued

		Nutrition standards for competitive foods sold in schools (includes items sold à la carte, in school stores and/or vending machines)			
State	Grade Level	Does the state have nutritional standards for competitive foods?	Max. calories from fat	Max. calories from saturated fat	Max. % of sugar by weight
Arkansas (cont.)	Middle and High Schools	No. However, portion size and nutrient standards to be released at a later date.	N/A	N/A	N/A

| Additional restrictions | Additional restrictions on vending machine | | | |
	Max. calories from fat, saturated fat, and sugar by weight	Restrictions on beverages sold in vending machines	Restrictions on access to vending machines	Notes
See restrictions under vending machines.	All FMNV and competitive foods and beverages, including sodas, are restricted to no more than 12 oz.	All FMNV and competitive foods and beverages, including sodas, are restricted to no more than 12 oz; the only exception to this rule is unsweetened, unflavored water. A choice of two fruits and/or 100% fruit juices must be offered for sale at the same time and place whenever competitive foods are sold. The standards require that at least 50% of the beverages made available for sale in vending machines and school stores be 100% fruit juice, low-fat or fat-free milk and unflavored, unsweetened water.	Any vending machine that contains FMNV must be closed during the meal service period if the machines are located in the food service area.	Middle, junior high, and high schools may not serve, provide access to, or award students with competitive foods or FMNVs until 30 minutes after the last lunch period.

continued

TABLE C-1 Continued

Nutrition standards for competitive foods sold in schools (includes items sold à la carte, in school stores and/or vending machines)

State	Grade Level	Does the state have nutritional standards for competitive foods?	Max. calories from fat	Max. calories from saturated fat	Max. % of sugar by weight
California	Elementary	Yes, the only food that may be sold to a pupil during breakfast and lunch periods is food that is sold as a full meal. This does not prohibit the sale of fruit, nonfried vegetables, legumes, beverages, dairy products, or grain products if they meet the outlined nutritional standards. Nutritional standards apply in elementary schools for those individual food items sold during morning or afternoon breaks.	35% for each individual food item. Does not include the sale of nuts, seeds, egg, cheese, legumes, and fruits and vegetables that have not been deep-fried.	10% for each individual food item's total calories may be from saturated fat. Does not include the sale of nuts, seeds, egg, cheese, legumes, and fruits and vegetables that have not been deep-fried.	35% of total weight for each individual food item. Does not include the sale of nuts, seeds, egg, cheese, legumes, and fruits and vegetables that have not been deep-fried.

Additional restrictions	Max. calories from fat, saturated fat, and sugar by weight	Restrictions on beverages sold in vending machines	Restrictions on access to vending machines	Notes
The only food that may be sold to a pupil during breakfast and lunch periods is food that is sold as a full meal. Individual items that meet the standards may be sold during morning or after-noon breaks. These items must meet the 35/10/35 restrictions and cannot exceed 250 calories per individual food item.	Allows for the sale of in-dividually sold dairy or whole grain food items if these items meet the 35/10/35 restric-tions and do not ex-ceed 175 calories per item.	The only beverages that may be sold in school vending machines are water, milk, and 100% fruit juices or fruit-based drinks that are at least 50% fruit juice with no added sweeteners.	None	An elementary school may permit the sale of food and beverage items that do not comply with the food nutrition standards as part of a school fund-raising event if the items are sold by pupils of the school and the sale of those items takes place off school premises and at least 30 minutes after the end of the school day.

(The column header "Additional restrictions on vending machine" spans the three columns: Max. calories from fat, saturated fat, and sugar by weight; Restrictions on beverages sold in vending machines; Restrictions on access to vending machines.)

continued

TABLE C-1 Continued

Nutrition standards for competitive foods sold in schools (includes items sold à la carte, in school stores and/or vending machines)

State	Grade Level	Does the state have nutritional standards for competitive foods?	Max. calories from fat	Max. calories from saturated fat	Max. % of sugar by weight
California (cont).	Middle and High Schools (Beginning July 1, 2007)	Yes. Requires all snacks sold outside of a USDA meal program to meet the 35/10/35 restrictions and cannot exceed 250 calories per individual food item with exemptions for nuts, seeds, egg, cheese, legumes, and fruits and vegetables that have not been deep-fried.	35% for each individual food item. Not to exceed 250 calories per individual food. Does not include the sale of nuts, seeds, egg, cheese, legumes, and fruits and vegetables that have not been deep-fried.	10% for each individual food item's total calories may be from saturated fat. Not to exceed 250 calories per individual food. Does not include the sale of nuts, seeds, egg, cheese, legumes, and fruits and vegetables that have not been deep-fried.	35% of total weight for each individual food item. Not to exceed 250 calories per individual food. Does not include the sale of nuts, seeds, egg, cheese, legumes, and fruits and vegetables that have not been deep-fried.

Additional restrictions	Max. calories from fat, saturated fat, and sugar by weight	Restrictions on beverages sold in vending machines	Restrictions on access to vending machines	Notes
	Additional restrictions on vending machine			
Prohibits entrée items sold outside of the USDA meal program from exceeding 400 calories and containing more than 4 g of fat per 100 calories per item.	Allows for the sale of individually sold dairy or whole grain food items if these items meet the 35/10/35 restrictions and do not exceed 250 calories per item.	By July 1, 2007, at least 50% of all beverages sold from 30 minutes before until 30 minutes after the school day must be: 1) Low- or nonfat milk or non dairy milk 2) Fruit and vegetable juices with at least 50% fruit or vegetable juice 3) Water 4) Electrolyte drinks with no more than 42 g of added sweetener per 20-oz serving. By July 1, 2009, all beverages sold to high school students must meet the above requirements.	Access to vending machines is restricted if products sold in vending machines do not meet nutritional guidelines. Products that do not comply with the nutritional guidelines may be available for sale no later than 30 minutes before the start of the school day and no sooner than 30 minutes after the end of the school day.	A middle or junior high school may permit the sale of beverages that do not comply with the state if the sale of those items meets all of the following criteria: 1) the sale occurs during a school-sponsored event and takes place at the location of the event at the end of the school day; and vending machines, pupil stores, and cafeterias are not used sooner than 30 minutes after the end of the school day.

continued

TABLE C-1 Continued

State	Grade Level	Nutrition standards for competitive foods sold in schools (includes items sold à la carte, in school stores and/or vending machines)			
		Does the state have nutritional standards for competitive foods?	Max. calories from fat	Max. calories from saturated fat	Max. % of sugar by weight
Colorado	Elementary, Middle, and High Schools	No	N/A	N/A	N/A

| | Additional restrictions on vending machine | | | |
Additional restrictions	Max. calories from fat, saturated fat, and sugar by weight	Restrictions on beverages sold in vending machines	Restrictions on access to vending machines	Notes
Competitive food service must be closed for a period beginning 30 minutes prior to and remain closed until 30 minutes after the last regular scheduled school lunch and/or school breakfast period on campus where these are served.	N/A	The restrictions of competitive food service can be waived for the service of competitive, mechanically vended beverages offered to students in high schools as long as federal rules or regulations for FMNV are not waived.	None	During the 2004 session, S.B. 103 was enacted requesting school districts to work with contractors to increase the nutritional value of food offered to students in school vending machines. School district boards of education were urged to adopt policies implementing a 50% threshold, meaning half of all vending machines shall offer healthy foods and beverages by the 2006-2007 school year.

continued

TABLE C-1 Continued

State	Grade Level	Does the state have nutritional standards for competitive foods?	Max. calories from fat	Max. calories from saturated fat	Max. % of sugar by weight
		Nutrition standards for competitive foods sold in schools (includes items sold à la carte, in school stores and/or vending machines)			
Connecticut	Elementary, Middle, and High Schools	Yes	18 g of fat per à la carte entrée	5 g (includes trans fat) of fat per à la carte entrée	15 g of sugar per à la carte entrée

Additional restrictions	Additional restrictions on vending machine			
	Max. calories from fat, saturated fat, and sugar by weight	Restrictions on beverages sold in vending machines	Restrictions on access to vending machines	Notes
All schools can only sell the following beverages, regardless of the source of the beverage: (1) Milk that may be flavored but contain no artificial sweeteners and no more than 4 g of sugar per oz, (2) nondairy milks such as soy or rice milk, which may be flavored but contain no artificial sweeteners, no more than 4 g of sugar per oz, no more than 35% of calories from fat per portion and no more than 10% of calories from saturated fat per portion, (3) 100% fruit juice, vegetable juice or combination of such juices, containing no added sugars, sweeteners or artificial sweeteners, (4) beverages that contain only water and fruit or vegetable juice and have no added sugars, sweeteners or artificial sweeteners, and (5) water, which may be flavored but contain no added sugars, sweeteners, artificial sweeteners or caffeine. Portion sizes of beverages, other than water, shall not exceed 12 oz. No school food authority shall permit the sale or dispensing to students of extra food items (candy) anywhere on the school premises from 30 minutes prior to the start of any state or federally subsidized milk or food service program until 30 minutes after such program.	N/A	See "additional restrictions"	See "additional restrictions"	Not later than August 1, 2006, and January 1 of each year thereafter, the Department of Education shall publish a set of nutrition standards for food items offered for sale to students at schools. During the 2004 legislative session, H.B. 5344 was enacted requiring each local and regional board of education to make available nutritious, low-fat foods and drinks for purchase by students. Low-fat dairy products and fresh or dried fruits should be made available for purchase at all times when food is available for purchase.

continued

TABLE C-1 Continued

		Nutrition standards for competitive foods sold in schools (includes items sold à la carte, in school stores and/or vending machines)			
State	Grade Level	Does the state have nutritional standards for competitive foods?	Max. calories from fat	Max. calories from saturated fat	Max. % of sugar by weight
Delaware	Elementary, Middle, and High Schools	No	N/A	N/A	N/A
District of Columbia	Elementary, Middle, and High Schools	No	N/A	N/A	N/A
Florida	Elementary, Middle, and High Schools	No	N/A	N/A	N/A

| | | Additional restrictions on vending machine | | |
Additional restrictions	Max. calories from fat, saturated fat, and sugar by weight	Restrictions on beverages sold in vending machines	Restrictions on access to vending machines	Notes
Each school district should implement a Child Nutrition Policy that minimally provides nutritious and balanced meals, purchasing practices that ensure the use of quality products, and adequate time to eat breakfast and lunch; Foods sold in addition to meals be selected to promote healthful eating habits and exclude those foods of minimal nutritional value.	N/A	None	None	Foods sold in addition to meals be selected to promote healthful eating habits and exclude those foods of minimal nutritional value.
No	N/A	None	None	None
FMNV may be sold in secondary schools only one hour following the close of the last lunch period.	N/A	A school board may allow the sale of carbonated beverages to high school students by a school activity or organization authorized by the principal if 100% fruit juice beverages are also offered at each location where carbonated beverages are sold. Non-carbonated beverages may be sold at all times during the day at any location.	None	State Board of Education requires district school food service program to adopt policies that control the sale of FMNV.

continued

TABLE C-1 Continued

		Nutrition standards for competitive foods sold in schools (includes items sold à la carte, in school stores and/or vending machines)			
State	Grade Level	Does the state have nutritional standards for competitive foods?	Max. calories from fat	Max. calories from saturated fat	Max. % of sugar by weight
Georgia	Elementary, Middle, and High Schools	No	N/A	N/A	N/A
Hawaii	Elementary	No	N/A	N/A	N/A

		Additional restrictions on vending machine		
Additional restrictions	Max. calories from fat, saturated fat, and sugar by weight	Restrictions on beverages sold in vending machines	Restrictions on access to vending machines	Notes
Prohibits the sale of FMNV in elementary schools from the beginning of the school day until that time when the last class/group of students eating lunch is scheduled to return to class.	N/A	Although not specific to vending machines, state policy prohibits the sale of FMNV in elementary schools from the beginning of the school day until that time when the last class/group of students eating lunch is scheduled to return to class.	Although not specific to vending machines, state policy prohibits the sale of FMNV in elementary schools from the beginning of the school day until that time when the last class/group of students eating lunch is scheduled to return to class.	None
The sale of food in all elementary and secondary schools shall be limited to the School Breakfast Program, School Lunch Program, milk, water, fruit and vegetable juice containing at least 50% fruit and/or vegetable.	N/A	N/A	N/A	Supplementary food sale policy indicates that only foods limited to the School Breakfast Program, School Lunch Program, milk, water, fruit and vegetable juice containing at least 50% fruit and/or vegetable shall be sold to elementary students.

continued

TABLE C-1 Continued

		Nutrition standards for competitive foods sold in schools (includes items sold à la carte, in school stores and/or vending machines)			
State	Grade Level	Does the state have nutritional standards for competitive foods?	Max. calories from fat	Max. calories from saturated fat	Max. % of sugar by weight
Hawaii (cont.)	Secondary schools	Yes. State places nutritional requirements on supplementary food and beverage items that can be sold during the meal periods.	25% of total calories	10% of total calories	25% of total calories, with the exception of fruits and vegetables.
Idaho	Elementary, Middle, and High Schools	No	N/A	N/A	N/A

	Additional restrictions on vending machine			
Additional restrictions	Max. calories from fat, saturated fat, and sugar by weight	Restrictions on beverages sold in vending machines	Restrictions on access to vending machines	Notes
Yes. Schools shall not permit the sale of other foods from the beginning of the school day to the end of the school day, except certain beverages through vending machines and supplementary food items. Also see notes.	No less than 50% fruit for all fruit juices.	80% of beverage selections from each vending machine at the schools shall be "healthy beverages," defined as milk, flavored milk, water, and fruit juice containing at least 50% juice, or other choices deemed appropriate by the Department of Education. The School Community Council and principal will determine the combination of beverages to be sold, including the remaining 20% of beverage selections, and shall have the discretion to ban caffeinated products. No alcoholic beverages, coffee, or coffee-based beverages may be dispensed.	Schools shall not permit the sale of other foods from the beginning of the school day to the end of the school day, except certain beverages through vending machines. Vending machines on elementary school campuses can only contain "healthy beverages."	The sale of food in all secondary schools shall be limited to the School Breakfast Program, School Lunch Program, milk, water, fruit and vegetable juice containing at least 50% fruit and/or vegetable, and other approved cafeteria supplementary food items. Students in secondary schools may be offered a wider variety of approved supplementary food and beverages during the meal period.
No	N/A	None	None	New Department of Education guidelines sent to districts "urge" schools to limit student access to unhealthy snacks and beverages.

continued

TABLE C-1 Continued

		Nutrition standards for competitive foods sold in schools (includes items sold à la carte, in school stores and/or vending machines)			
State	Grade Level	Does the state have nutritional standards for competitive foods?	Max. calories from fat	Max. calories from saturated fat	Max. % of sugar by weight
Illinois	Elementary	Yes	35%	10%	35%

| | | Additional restrictions on vending machine | | |
Additional restrictions	Max. calories from fat, saturated fat, and sugar by weight	Restrictions on beverages sold in vending machines	Restrictions on access to vending machines	Notes
Exceptions to fat and sugar standards include nuts, seeds, nut butters, egg, cheese packaged for individual sale, fruits or non-fried vegetables, or low-fat yogurt products; students may only be served the following beverages: flavored or plain whole, reduced fat (2%), low-fat (1%), or nonfat fluid milk that meets state and local standards for pasteurized fluid milk; reduced fat and enriched alternative dairy beverages (i.e., rice, nut, or soy milk, or any other alternative dairy beverage approved by the U.S. Department of Agriculture [USDA]); fruit and vegetable drinks containing 50% or more fruit or vegetable juice; water (non-flavored, non-sweetened, and non-carbonated); fruit smoothie (yogurt or ice based) that contains less than 400 calories and no added sugars, and is made from fresh or frozen fruit or fruit drinks that contain at least 50% fruit juice; and any beverage exempted from the USDA's list of Foods of Minimal Nutritional Value.	N/A	Students may only be served the following beverages: flavored or plain whole, reduced fat (2%), low-fat (1%), or nonfat fluid milk that meets state and local standards for pasteurized fluid milk; reduced fat and enriched alternative dairy beverages (i.e., rice, nut, or soy milk, or any other alternative dairy beverage approved by the U.S. Department of Agriculture [USDA]); fruit and vegetable drinks containing 50% or more fruit or vegetable juice; water (non-flavored, non-sweetened, and non-carbonated); fruit smoothie (yogurt or ice based) that contains less than 400 calories and no added sugars, and is made from fresh or frozen fruit or fruit drinks that contain at least 50% fruit juice; and any beverage exempted from the USDA's list of Foods of Minimal Nutritional Value.	None	Identifies "competitive foods" to include all confections, candy, potato chips, carbonated beverages, fruit drinks containing less than 50% fruit juice, tea, coffee and any other food item designated as such by the State Board of Education.

continued

TABLE C-1 Continued

| State | Grade Level | Nutrition standards for competitive foods sold in schools (includes items sold à la carte, in school stores and/or vending machines) | | | |
		Does the state have nutritional standards for competitive foods?	Max. calories from fat	Max. calories from saturated fat	Max. % of sugar by weight
Illinois (cont.)	Middle and High Schools	Yes	35%	10%	35%

| Additional restrictions | Additional restrictions on vending machine | | | |
	Max. calories from fat, saturated fat, and sugar by weight	Restrictions on beverages sold in vending machines	Restrictions on access to vending machines	Notes
Exceptions to fat and sugar standards include nuts, seeds, nut butters, egg, cheese packaged for individual sale, fruits or non-fried vegetables, or low-fat yogurt products; students may only be served the following beverages: flavored or plain whole, reduced fat (2%), low-fat (1%), or nonfat fluid milk that meets state and local standards for pasteurized fluid milk; reduced fat and enriched alternative dairy beverages (i.e., rice, nut, or soy milk, or any other alternative dairy beverage approved by the U.S. Department of Agriculture [USDA]); fruit and vegetable drinks containing 50% or more fruit or vegetable juice; water (non-flavored, non-sweetened, and non-carbonated); fruit smoothie (yogurt or ice based) that contains less than 400 calories and no added sugars, and is made from fresh or frozen fruit or fruit drinks that contain at least 50% fruit juice; and any beverage exempted from the USDA's list of Foods of Minimal Nutritional Value.	N/A	Students may only be served the following beverages: flavored or plain whole, reduced fat (2%), low-fat (1%), or nonfat fluid milk that meets state and local standards for pasteurized fluid milk; reduced fat and enriched alternative dairy beverages (i.e., rice, nut, or soy milk, or any other alternative dairy beverage approved by the U.S. Department of Agriculture [USDA]); fruit and vegetable drinks containing 50% or more fruit or vegetable juice; water (non-flavored, non-sweetened, and non-carbonated); fruit smoothie (yogurt or ice based) that contains less than 400 calories and no added sugars, and is made from fresh or frozen fruit or fruit drinks that contain at least 50% fruit juice; and any beverage exempted from the USDA's list of Foods of Minimal Nutritional Value.	None	Local school authorities for junior and senior high schools shall establish such instructions as are desired to regulate the sale of competitive foods to students during the time period designated by local school authorities as the regular breakfast and lunch periods.

continued

TABLE C-1 Continued

State	Grade Level	Does the state have nutritional standards for competitive foods?	Max. calories from fat	Max. calories from saturated fat	Max. % of sugar by weight
		Nutrition standards for competitive foods sold in schools (includes items sold à la carte, in school stores and/or vending machines)			
Indiana	Elementary, Middle, and High Schools	No	30% for a "better choice food"	10% for a "better choice food"	35% for a "better choice food"
Iowa	Elementary, Middle, and High Schools	No	N/A	N/A	N/A

| Additional restrictions | Additional restrictions on vending machine | | | |
	Max. calories from fat, saturated fat, and sugar by weight	Restrictions on beverages sold in vending machines	Restrictions on access to vending machines	Notes
At least 50% of the food items available for sale at a school or on school grounds must qualify as "better choice foods" and at least 50% of the beverage items available for sale at a school or on school grounds must qualify as "better choice beverages." A food item available for sale at a school or on school grounds may not exceed the following portion limits if the food item contains more than 210 calories: (1) In the case of potato chips, crackers, popcorn, cereal, trail mixes, nuts, seeds, dried fruit, and jerky, 1.75 oz (2) In the case of cookies and cereal bars, 2 oz (3) In the case of bakery items, including pastries, muffins, and doughnuts, 3 oz (4) In the case of frozen desserts, including ice cream, 3 fl oz (5) In the case of nonfrozen yogurt, 8 oz (6) In the case of entrée items and side dish items, including french fries and onion rings, the food item available for sale may not exceed the portion of the same entrée item or side dish item that is served as part of the school lunch program or school breakfast program. A beverage item available for sale at a school or on school grounds may not exceed 20 oz.	N/A	N/A	Elementary students may not have access to vending machines.	None
No	N/A	N/A	None	Stricter standards would be set by local school district policy.

continued

TABLE C-1 Continued

State	Grade Level	Nutrition standards for competitive foods sold in schools (includes items sold à la carte, in school stores and/or vending machines)			
		Does the state have nutritional standards for competitive foods?	Max. calories from fat	Max. calories from saturated fat	Max. % of sugar by weight
Kansas	Elementary, Middle, and High Schools	No (see notes)	N/A	N/A	N/A

	Additional restrictions on vending machine			
Additional restrictions	Max. calories from fat, saturated fat, and sugar by weight	Restrictions on beverages sold in vending machines	Restrictions on access to vending machines	Notes
No	N/A	None	None	Legislation enacted in 2005 required the State Board of Education to develop nutrition guidelines for all foods and beverages sold during the school day. Schools must consider the recommendations released by the board when developing their wellness policies. Schools are not required to adopt standards.

continued

TABLE C-1 Continued

State	Grade Level	Nutrition standards for competitive foods sold in schools (includes items sold à la carte, in school stores and/or vending machines)			
		Does the state have nutritional standards for competitive foods?	Max. calories from fat	Max. calories from saturated fat	Max. % of sugar by weight
Kentucky	Elementary, Middle, and High Schools	Yes	Food items may not contain more than 30% of calories from total fat, excluding nuts and seeds.	10% of calories from saturated fat	32% sugar by weight (includes natural and added sugars)

| Additional restrictions | Additional restrictions on vending machine | | | |
	Max. calories from fat, saturated fat, and sugar by weight	Restrictions on beverages sold in vending machines	Restrictions on access to vending machines	Notes
Sale of competitive foods and beverages is prohibited from the arrival of the first student at the school building until 30 minutes after the last lunch period, except for any food or beverage item sold à la carte. Pastas, meats and soups may not contain more than 450 mg of sodium per serving. Pizza, sandwiches and main dishes may not contain more than 600 mg per serving. Chips, cereals, crackers, baked goods and other snack items may not contain more than 300 mg of sodium per serving. Portion sizes for cookies shall not exceed one oz. Portion sizes for non-frozen yogurt may not exceed eight oz and for frozen dessert items, including low-fat or fat-free ice cream, frozen fruit juice bars and frozen real fruit items may not exceed four oz.	Chips, cereals, crackers, baked goods and other snack items may not contain more than 300 mg of sodium per serving. Portion sizes for chips, crackers, popcorn, cereal, trail mix, nuts, seeds, jerky, cereal bars, granola bars, pastries, muffins, doughnuts, bagels and other bakery-type items may not exceed two oz. Portion sizes for cookies shall not exceed one oz.	Only "school-day-approved beverages" are allowed, defined as water, 100% fruit juice, low-fat milk and any other beverage containing no more than 10 g of sugar per serving, to be sold in elementary school vending machines, school stores, canteens or fund-raisers during the school day. 17 oz maximum sized beverage for elementary students, 20 oz maximum for middle and high school students.	Sale of competitive foods and beverages is prohibited from the arrival of the first student at the school building until 30 minutes after the last lunch period.	Affected items are defined as any food or beverage item sold in competition with the National School Breakfast and Lunch program except those sold à la carte.

continued

TABLE C-1 Continued

		Nutrition standards for competitive foods sold in schools (includes items sold à la carte, in school stores and/or vending machines)			
State	Grade Level	Does the state have nutritional standards for competitive foods?	Max. calories from fat	Max. calories from saturated fat	Max. % of sugar by weight
Louisiana	Elementary Schools	Yes	35%, with the exception of un-sweetened seeds or nuts.	N/A	30 g of sugar per serving.

| | Additional restrictions on vending machine | | | |
Additional restrictions	Max. calories from fat, saturated fat, and sugar by weight	Restrictions on beverages sold in vending machines	Restrictions on access to vending machines	Notes
Yes. Sale of FMNVs and snacks and desserts that exceed 150 calories per serving are prohibited. Fresh pastries cannot be sold on school grounds.	Sale of FMNVs and snacks and desserts that exceed 150 calories per serving and fat restrictions are prohibited.	Prohibited from selling beverages that exceed 16 oz from 30 minutes before the start of the school day until 30 minutes after the day ends. Exceptions: milk, water, and fruit juices that are composed of 100% fruit or vegetable juice.	No access before the end of the last lunch period (see notes).	Reimbursement for lunch, special milk, and/or breakfast may be withheld from schools if concessions, canteens, snack bars, or vending machines are operated on a profit basis before the end of the last lunch period.

continued

TABLE C-1 Continued

State	Grade Level	Nutrition standards for competitive foods sold in schools (includes items sold à la carte, in school stores and/or vending machines)			
		Does the state have nutritional standards for competitive foods?	Max. calories from fat	Max. calories from saturated fat	Max. % of sugar by weight
Louisiana (cont.)	Middle and High Schools	Yes	35%, with the exception of unsweetened seeds or nuts.	N/A	30 g of sugar per serving.

| | Additional restrictions on vending machine | | | |
Additional restrictions	Max. calories from fat, saturated fat, and sugar by weight	Restrictions on beverages sold in vending machines	Restrictions on access to vending machines	Notes
Yes. Sale of FMNVs and snacks and desserts that exceed 150 calories per serving are prohibited. Fresh pastries cannot be sold on school grounds.	Sale of FMNVs and snacks and desserts that exceed 150 calories per serving and fat restrictions are prohibited.	Prohibited from selling beverages that exceed 16 oz from 30 minutes before the start of the school day until 30 minutes after the day ends. Food service program must ensure that milk, water, and fruit and vegetable juices make up at least 50% of the beverages available to students and that no more than 50% of the available food items exceed the requirements.	No access before the last 10 minutes of each lunch period (see notes).	Reimbursement for lunch, special breakfast may be withheld from schools if concessions, canteens, snack bars, or vending machines are operated on a profit basis before the last 10 minutes of each lunch period. In grades 7–12 with multiple lunch periods, concessions, canteens, snack bars, vending machines or other food sales between lunch periods are allowed if the following guidelines are implemented: no food item shall be sold before the last 10 minutes of each lunch period, lunch periods shall be divided by a period of time so there is no interaction between students of different lunch periods, and students can't have access to competitive foods before the last 10 minutes of each lunch period.

continued

TABLE C-1 Continued

State	Grade Level	Nutrition standards for competitive foods sold in schools (includes items sold à la carte, in school stores and/or vending machines)			
		Does the state have nutritional standards for competitive foods?	Max. calories from fat	Max. calories from saturated fat	Max. % of sugar by weight
Maine	Elementary, Middle, and High Schools	Yes	N/A	N/A	N/A
Maryland	Elementary, Middle, and High Schools	No; however, state prohibits the sale of FMNV from 12:01 am until the end of the last lunch period anywhere in the school.	N/A	N/A	N/A
Massachusetts	Elementary, Middle, and High Schools	No	N/A	N/A	N/A

Additional restrictions	Max. calories from fat, saturated fat, and sugar by weight	Restrictions on beverages sold in vending machines	Restrictions on access to vending machines	Notes
The sale of foods of minimal nutritional value is prohibited. This policy effectively eliminates all sodas, candy, gum, and many high-calorie snack sales in vending machines and school stores.	N/A	The sale of foods of minimal nutritional value is prohibited. This policy effectively eliminates all sodas, candy, gum, and many high-calorie snack sales in vending machines and school stores.	None	Any food or beverage sold during the school day of a school participating in the National School Lunch or Breakfast Program must be a planned part of the total food service program. Only items that contribute to both the nutritional needs of children and development of desirable food habits will be sold. Food service program must post caloric information for prepackaged à la carte menu items at the point-of-decision.
None	N/A	None	All vending machines in public schools must have and use a timing device to automatically prohibit or allow access in accordance with nutrition policies established by local county boards of education by August 1, 2006.	None
None	N/A	None	None	None

continued

TABLE C-1 Continued

State	Grade Level	Nutrition standards for competitive foods sold in schools (includes items sold à la carte, in school stores and/or vending machines)			
		Does the state have nutritional standards for competitive foods?	Max. calories from fat	Max. calories from saturated fat	Max. % of sugar by weight
Michigan	Elementary, Middle, and High Schools	No	N/A	N/A	N/A
Minnesota	Elementary, Middle, and High Schools	No	N/A	N/A	N/A
Mississippi	Elementary, Middle, and High Schools	No	N/A	N/A	N/A
Missouri	Elementary, Middle, and High Schools	No	N/A	N/A	N/A

| Additional restrictions | Max. calories from fat, saturated fat, and sugar by weight | Additional restrictions on vending machine | | Notes |
		Restrictions on beverages sold in vending machines	Restrictions on access to vending machines	
No	N/A	None	None	State Board of Education recommends that each school building offer and promote certain food and beverages offered outside the federal school meal program.
No	N/A	None	None	None
School food services may only sell those foods that are components of the approved federal meal pattern being served, with the exception of milk. A student may purchase individual components of a meal only if a full meal was also purchased. Also see notes.	N/A	None	Although not specific to vending machines, state policy indicates that no food is to be sold on campus for one hour before breakfast or one hour before lunch and until the end of either serving period. Any food may be sold after breakfast, until one hour before lunch, and any time after the end of the last lunch period.	The state policy is a minimum requirement; local school boards are allowed to adopt more restrictive policies. Waivers to the state policy may be granted in school districts where high school and elementary schools are in the same building/center. If a waiver is granted, schools must ensure that only high school students have access to vending machines and that access shall be limited starting one hour prior to the high school's meal service and during the meal service.
No	N/A	None	None	None

continued

TABLE C-1 Continued

		Nutrition standards for competitive foods sold in schools (includes items sold à la carte, in school stores and/or vending machines)			
State	Grade Level	Does the state have nutritional standards for competitive foods?	Max. calories from fat	Max. calories from saturated fat	Max. % of sugar by weight
Montana	Elementary, Middle, and High Schools	No	N/A	N/A	N/A
Nebraska	Elementary, Middle, and High Schools	No, see notes	N/A	N/A	N/A

| Additional restrictions | Additional restrictions on vending machine | | | |
	Max. calories from fat, saturated fat, and sugar by weight	Restrictions on beverages sold in vending machines	Restrictions on access to vending machines	Notes
No	N/A	None	None	None
No Foods of Minimal Nutritional Value, as defined by the USDA, can be sold in the Food Service areas beginning 1/2 hr before breakfast and/or lunch service until 1/2 hr after meal service under any circumstances. The sale of any foods in competition with the National School Lunch and School Breakfast Program is prohibited anywhere on school/institution premises during the period beginning 30 minutes prior to the serving period for breakfast and/or lunch and lasting until 30 minutes after the serving of breakfast and/or lunch, unless all proceeds earned during these time periods go to the school nutrition program.	N/A	None	None	No Foods of Minimal Nutritional Value, as defined by the USDA, can be sold in the Food Service Areas beginning 1/2 hr before breakfast and/or lunch service until 1/2 hr after meal service under any circumstances. The sale of any foods in competition with the National School Lunch and School Breakfast Program is prohibited anywhere on school/institution premises during the period beginning 30 minutes prior to the serving period for breakfast and/or lunch and lasting until 30 minutes after the serving of breakfast and/or lunch, unless all proceeds earned during these time periods go to the school nutrition program.

continued

TABLE C-1 Continued

State	Grade Level	Nutrition standards for competitive foods sold in schools (includes items sold à la carte, in school stores and/or vending machines)			
		Does the state have nutritional standards for competitive foods?	Max. calories from fat	Max. calories from saturated fat	Max. % of sugar by weight
Nevada	Elementary, Middle, and High Schools	No	N/A	N/A	N/A
New Hampshire	Elementary, Middle, and High Schools	No	N/A	N/A	N/A
New Jersey	Elementary, Middle, and High Schools	Yes	No more than 8 g of total fat per serving, with the exception of nuts and seeds	No more than 2 g of saturated fat per serving	Not specified

| Additional restrictions | Additional restrictions on vending machine | | | Notes |
	Max. calories from fat, saturated fat, and sugar by weight	Restrictions on beverages sold in vending machines	Restrictions on access to vending machines	
No	N/A	None	None	Some local school districts have initiated stricter requirements; no state mandate. Department of Education released nutrition guidelines to assist schools in drafting local school wellness policies.
None	N/A	None	None	Within the parameters of the federal law, schools create their own policies around foods sold and eaten within a school day.
Prohibits the following items from being sold in elementary, middle and high schools: foods of minimal nutritional value, all food and beverage items listing sugar, in any form, as the first ingredient, and all forms of candy. Beverages sold to students cannot exceed 12 oz with the exception of water and 2% milk; servings of whole milk cannot exceed 8 oz. In elementary schools, the only beverages that can be sold include milk, water or 100% fruit or vegetable juices. At least 60% of the beverages offered in middle and high schools, other than milk and water, must be 100% fruit or vegetable juices.	See restrictions under competitive foods.	Beverages sold to students cannot exceed 12 oz with the exception of water and 2% milk; servings of whole milk cannot exceed 8 oz. In elementary schools, the only beverages that can be sold include milk, water or 100% fruit or vegetable juices. At least 60% of the beverages offered in middle and high schools, other than milk and water, must be 100% fruit or vegetable juices.	None	School districts must adopt a school nutrition policy, and a year later, schools will have to adapt their policies to the model policy released by the Department of Agriculture. The model policy requirements were outlined in this chart.

continued

TABLE C-1 Continued

		Nutrition standards for competitive foods sold in schools (includes items sold à la carte, in school stores and/or vending machines)			
State	Grade Level	Does the state have nutritional standards for competitive foods?	Max. calories from fat	Max. calories from saturated fat	Max. % of sugar by weight
New Mexico	Elementary schools	Yes	N/A	N/A	N/A

| Additional restrictions | Additional restrictions on vending machine | | | |
	Max. calories from fat, saturated fat, and sugar by weight	Restrictions on beverages sold in vending machines	Restrictions on access to vending machines	Notes
Vending machines may only contain milk with a fat content of 2% or less, soy milk, or water. Vending machines may not sell food products. Restrictions on à la carte items are similar to those on items in vending machines (see Section 6.12.5 of NMAC).	N/A	Vending machines may only contain milk with a fat content of 2% or less, soy milk, or water.	Beverages sold in vending machines to students in elementary schools shall only be sold after the last lunch period is completed.	Carbonated beverages and any food products may not be sold in vending machines at elementary schools.

continued

TABLE C-1 Continued

		Nutrition standards for competitive foods sold in schools (includes items sold à la carte, in school stores and/or vending machines)			
State	Grade Level	Does the state have nutritional standards for competitive foods?	Max. calories from fat	Max. calories from saturated fat	Max. % of sugar by weight
New Mexico (cont.)	Middle schools	Yes	N/A	N/A	N/A

| Additional restrictions | Additional restrictions on vending machine | | | |
	Max. calories from fat, saturated fat, and sugar by weight	Restrictions on beverages sold in vending machines	Restrictions on access to vending machines	Notes
Food products sold in vending machines to students in middle schools are subject to the following requirements: (i) Nuts, seeds, cheese, yogurt, and fruit may be sold in vending machines in middle schools at any time and are not subject to the restrictions in item (ii) of this subparagraph. (ii) Food products other than those listed in item (i) of this subparagraph shall only be sold after the last lunch period is completed and are subject to the following restrictions: shall contain no more than 200 calories per container or per package or amount served and shall contain no more than 8 g of fat per container or per package or amount served with no more than 2 g of fat from saturated and trans fats and shall contain no more than 15 g of sugar per package or amount served. Restrictions on à la carte items are similar to those on items in vending machines (see Section 6.12.5 of NMAC).	N/A	Vending machines may only contain milk with a fat content of 2% or less, soy milk, water, or 100% fruit juice that has no added sweeteners and no more that 125 calories per container and a serving size not to exceed 20 oz.	N/A	Food products sold in vending machines to students in middle schools are subject to the following requirements: (i) Nuts, seeds, cheese, yogurt, and fruit may be sold in vending machines in middle schools at any time and are not subject to the restrictions in item (ii) of this subparagraph. (ii) Food products other than those listed in item (i) of this subparagraph shall only be sold after the last lunch period is completed and are subject to the following restrictions: shall contain no more than 200 calories per container or per package or amount served and shall contain no more than 8 g of fat per container or per package or amount served with no more than 2 g of fat from saturated and trans fats and shall contain no more than 15 g of sugar per package or amount served.

continued

TABLE C-1 Continued

State	Grade Level	Nutrition standards for competitive foods sold in schools (includes items sold à la carte, in school stores and/or vending machines)			
		Does the state have nutritional standards for competitive foods?	Max. calories from fat	Max. calories from saturated fat	Max. % of sugar by weight
New Mexico (cont.)	High schools	Yes	N/A	N/A	N/A

Additional restrictions	Additional restrictions on vending machine			
	Max. calories from fat, saturated fat, and sugar by weight	Restrictions on beverages sold in vending machines	Restrictions on access to vending machines	Notes
Food products sold in vending machines to students in high schools may be sold at any time subject to the following requirements: Nuts, seeds, cheese, yogurt, and fruit may be sold in vending machines in high schools at any time and are not subject to the restrictions in item (ii) of this subparagraph. (ii) Food products other than those listed in item (i) of this subparagraph are subject to the following restrictions: shall contain no more than 200 calories per container or per package or amount served and shall contain no more than 8 g of fat per container or per package or amount served with no more than 2 g of fat from saturated and trans fats and shall contain no more than 15 g of sugar per container or per package or amount served. Restrictions on à la carte items are similar to those on items in vending machines (see Section 6.12.5 of NMAC).		Vending machines may only contain milk with a fat content of 2% or less, soy milk, water, or juice that is at least 50% fruit and that has no added sweeteners and a serving size not to exceed 20 oz.	The following beverages may only be sold in vending machines after the last lunch period is completed: carbonated soft drinks that are both sugar free and caffeine free; non-carbonated flavored water with no added sweeteners; and sports drinks.	Food products sold in vending machines to students in high schools may be sold at any time subject to the following requirements: (i) Nuts, seeds, cheese, yogurt, and fruit may be sold in vending machines in high schools at any time and are not subject to the restrictions in item (ii) of this subparagraph.(ii) Food products other than those listed in item (i) of this subparagraph are subject to the following restrictions: shall contain no more than 200 calories per container or per package or amount served and shall contain no more than 8 g of fat per container or per package or amount served with no more than 2 g of fat from saturated and trans fats and shall contain no more than 15 g of sugar per container or per package or amount served.

continued

TABLE C-1 Continued

State	Grade Level	Nutrition standards for competitive foods sold in schools (includes items sold à la carte, in school stores and/or vending machines)			
		Does the state have nutritional standards for competitive foods?	Max. calories from fat	Max. calories from saturated fat	Max. % of sugar by weight
New York	Elementary, Middle, and High Schools	No	N/A	N/A	N/A
North Carolina	Elementary schools	Yes (see notes)	Not specified	Not specified	Not specified

| | Additional restrictions on vending machine | | | |
Additional restrictions	Max. calories from fat, saturated fat, and sugar by weight	Restrictions on beverages sold in vending machines	Restrictions on access to vending machines	Notes
From the beginning of the school day until the end of the last scheduled meal period, no sweetened soda water, no chewing gum, no candy including hard candy, jellies, gums, marshmallow candies, fondant, licorice, spun candy and candy coated popcorn, and no water ices except those which contain fruit or fruit juices, shall be sold in any public school within the state.	N/A	Although not specific to vending machines, state policy prohibits sale of sweetened soda water from the beginning of the school day until the end of the last scheduled meal period.	Although not specific to vending machines, state policy prohibits sale of sweetened soda water from the beginning of the school day until the end of the last scheduled meal period.	None
Schools may not sell soft drinks to students at elementary schools.	Prohibits snack vending.	Schools may not sell soft drinks to students at elementary schools.	None	The State Board of Education is required to develop nutrition standards for school meals, à la carte food and beverage items and after-school snack program (all grades). The standards must promote an increase in fruits, vegetables, and whole-grain products and decrease foods high in fat and sugar (all grades). Implementation of the standards in elementary schools must be achieved by the 2007-2008 school year, followed by middle and high schools.

continued

TABLE C-1 Continued

		Nutrition standards for competitive foods sold in schools (includes items sold à la carte, in school stores and/or vending machines)			
State	Grade Level	Does the state have nutritional standards for competitive foods?	Max. calories from fat	Max. calories from saturated fat	Max. % of sugar by weight
North Carolina (cont.)	Secondary schools	Yes (see notes)	Not specified	Not specified	Not specified
North Dakota	Elementary, Middle, and High Schools	No	N/A	N/A	N/A
Ohio	Elementary, Middle, and High Schools	No	N/A	N/A	N/A
Oklahoma	Elementary, Middle, and High Schools	No; however, elementary school students cannot have access to FMNVs except on special occasions. Middle and junior high school students do not have access to FMNVs except after school, at evening events, and on special occasions.	N/A	N/A	N/A

| Additional restrictions | Additional restrictions on vending machine | | | |
	Max. calories from fat, saturated fat, and sugar by weight	Restrictions on beverages sold in vending machines	Restrictions on access to vending machines	Notes
Soft drinks may not be sold to students until after the end of the last lunch period with the approval of the local school board of education.	75% of snack vending products offered in middle and high schools to not exceed 200 calories per portion or package.	Sales of sugared, carbonated soft drinks in middle school vending machines are prohibited. Offering of sugared carbonated soft drinks in high school vending machines cannot be more than 50% of the total items for sale. Bottled water products must be available in every school with beverage vending.	Sale of soft drinks during breakfast and lunch periods in middle and high schools is prohibited.	
No	N/A	None	None	None
No	N/A	None	None	State law requires public school districts to pass and enforce a local Food For Sale Policy through board resolution.
Middle and junior high school students do not have access to FMNVs except after school, at evening events, and on special occasions, with the exception of diet sodas with less than ten calories per serving.	N/A	Middle and junior high school students do not have access to FMNVs except after school, at evening events, and on special occasions, with the exception of diet sodas with less than ten calories per serving.	None	High school students must have access to healthy food choices. Incentives, such as lower prices, should be provided to encourage selection of healthy food choices over FMNVs.

continued

TABLE C-1 Continued

		Nutrition standards for competitive foods sold in schools (includes items sold à la carte, in school stores and/or vending machines)			
State	Grade Level	Does the state have nutritional standards for competitive foods?	Max. calories from fat	Max. calories from saturated fat	Max. % of sugar by weight
Oregon	Elementary, Middle, and High Schools	No (see notes)	N/A	N/A	N/A
Pennsylvania	Elementary, Middle, and High Schools	No	N/A	N/A	N/A

	Additional restrictions on vending machine			
Additional restrictions	Max. calories from fat, saturated fat, and sugar by weight	Restrictions on beverages sold in vending machines	Restrictions on access to vending machines	Notes
No	N/A	None	None	If approved by a school board, FMNV may be sold outside the food service area during breakfast or lunch periods, and may be offered in an offer vs serve program.
No	N/A	None	None	None

continued

TABLE C-1 Continued

		Nutrition standards for competitive foods sold in schools (includes items sold à la carte, in school stores and/or vending machines)			
State	Grade Level	Does the state have nutritional standards for competitive foods?	Max. calories from fat	Max. calories from saturated fat	Max. % of sugar by weight
Rhode Island	Elementary, Middle, and High Schools	No	N/A	N/A	N/A

| Additional restrictions | Additional restrictions on vending machine | | | |
	Max. calories from fat, saturated fat, and sugar by weight	Restrictions on beverages sold in vending machines	Restrictions on access to vending machines	Notes
All elementary, middle, and junior high schools can only offer healthier beverages and snacks. Healthier beverages are defined as: (1) Water, including carbonated water, flavored or sweetened with 100% fruit juice and containing no added sweetener; (2) 2% fat milk, 1% fat milk, nonfat milk, and dairy alternatives, such as fortified soy beverages, plain or flavored, with a sugar content of not more than 4 g per oz; (3) 100% fruit juice or fruit based drinks that are composed of no less than 50% fruit juice and have no added sweetener; and (4) Vegetable-based drinks that are composed of no less than 50% vegetable juice and have no added sweetener. Healthier snacks are defined as: (1) Individually sold portions of nuts, nut butters, seeds, egg and cheese packaged for individual sale, fruit, vegetables that have not been deep-fried and legumes; (2) Individually sold portions of low-fat yogurt with not more than 4 g of total carbohydrates per oz and reduced fat or low fat cheese packaged for individual sale; and (3) Individually sold enriched or fortified grain or grain products or whole grain foods that contain no more than 30% calories from fat, no more than 10% total calories from saturated fat, and no more than 7 g of total sugar per oz.	N/A	All elementary, middle, and junior high schools can only offer healthier beverages and snacks. Healthier beverages are defined as: (1) Water, including carbonated water, flavored or sweetened with 100% fruit juice and containing no added sweetener; (2) 2% fat milk, 1% fat milk, nonfat milk, and dairy alternatives, such as fortified soy beverages, plain or flavored, with a sugar content of not more than 4 g per oz; (3) 100% fruit juice or fruit based drinks that are composed of no less than 50% fruit juice and have no added sweetener; and (4) Vegetable-based drinks that are composed of no less than 50% vegetable juice and have no added sweetener. Healthier snacks are defined as: (1) Individually sold portions of nuts, nut butters, seeds, egg and cheese packaged for individual sale, fruit, vegetables that have not been deep-fried and legumes; (2) Individually sold portions of low-fat yogurt with not more than 4 g of total carbohydrates per oz and reduced fat or low fat cheese packaged for individual sale; and (3) Individually sold enriched or fortified grain or grain products or whole grain foods that contain no more than 30% calories from fat, no more than 10% total calories from saturated fat, and no more than 7 g of total sugar per oz.	None	None

continued

TABLE C-1 Continued

State	Grade Level	Nutrition standards for competitive foods sold in schools (includes items sold à la carte, in school stores and/or vending machines)			
		Does the state have nutritional standards for competitive foods?	Max. calories from fat	Max. calories from saturated fat	Max. % of sugar by weight
South Carolina	Elementary, Middle, and High Schools	No	N/A	N/A	N/A
South Dakota	Elementary, Middle, and High Schools	No	N/A	N/A	N/A

| Additional restrictions | Additional restrictions on vending machine | | | |
	Max. calories from fat, saturated fat, and sugar by weight	Restrictions on beverages sold in vending machines	Restrictions on access to vending machines	Notes
No	N/A	None	None	Each school district must establish a Co-ordinated School Health Advisory Council (CSHAC) responsible for assessing, planning, implementing and monitoring school health policies and programs. The CSHAC is responsible for determining which snacks may be sold in vending machines in elementary schools. Each school board of trustees must establish restrictions on food and beverage items made available through vending machines.
No	N/A	None	None	None

continued

TABLE C-1 Continued

State	Grade Level	Nutrition standards for competitive foods sold in schools (includes items sold à la carte, in school stores and/or vending machines)			
		Does the state have nutritional standards for competitive foods?	Max. calories from fat	Max. calories from saturated fat	Max. % of sugar by weight
Tennessee	Pre-K, Elementary, and Middle Schools	Yes	35% excluding nuts, seeds, and nut butters.	At or below 10%	35%
Tennessee (cont.)	High School	No	N/A	N/A	N/A

| | Additional restrictions on vending machine | | | |
| | | | | |

Additional restrictions	Max. calories from fat, saturated fat, and sugar by weight	Restrictions on beverages sold in vending machines	Restrictions on access to vending machines	Notes
Portion size for à la carte entrées cannot exceed the portion size of comparable portions offered as part of school meals. Chips, cereals, crackers, french fries, baked goods, and other snack items cannot contain more than 230 mg of sodium per serving. Pastas, meats, and soups may not contain more than 480 mg of sodium per serving. Pizza, sandwiches, and main dishes may not contain more than 600 mg of sodium per serving. Portion size restrictions: for cookies (1 oz); for baked goods (2 oz); chips, crackers, popcorn, cereal, trail mix, nuts, seeds, dried fruit or jerky (1 1/4 oz); frozen dessert (4 oz); frozen yogurt (8 oz). Pure cheese can only be sold in 1 oz sizes and cannot exceed 3.5 g of fat. See beverage restrictions under vending machine column.	Same restrictions as provided under "competitive foods."	Only beverages that can be sold include: reduced fat, low-fat, or skim milk or USDA approved alternative dairy beverages; 100% fruit juice; non-flavored, non-sweetened, non-caffeinated water; and low-calorie non-carbonated beverages containing no additional sweeteners and no more than 15 calories per serving. Beverages sold cannot exceed 8 oz, with the exception of non-flavored water.	None	These standards do not apply to foods served as a federally reimbursable meal; however, the Board strongly recommends that school meal programs meet the standards. An individual food item that is part of the day's reimbursable school lunch program may be sold as an à la carte item and does not need to comply to the nutritional standards.
None	N/A	None	None	None

continued

TABLE C-1 Continued

		Nutrition standards for competitive foods sold in schools (includes items sold à la carte, in school stores and/or vending machines)			
State	Grade Level	Does the state have nutritional standards for competitive foods?	Max. calories from fat	Max. calories from saturated fat	Max. % of sugar by weight
Texas	Elementary (defined through grade 6)	Yes	Schools and other vendors may not serve food items containing more than 28 g of fat per serving size more than twice per week. By the 2006-07 school year, the goal is to reduce this to 23 g of fat. French fries and other fried potato products must not exceed 3 oz per serving and may not be offered more than once per week and students may only purchase one serving at a time. Schools serving potato chips should use reduced fat, no more than 5 g per oz, or baked varieties when possible. Beginning in 2006-07 school year, schools should reduce the purchase of any products containing trans fats. Schools also must abide by maximum portion sizes outlined in the Texas Public School Nutrition Policy.	Not specified	Unflavored or flavored milks and beverages may not contain more than 30 g total sugar per 8 oz serving. Frozen fruit slushes must contain a minimum of 50% fruit juice.

Additional restrictions	Max. calories from fat, saturated fat, and sugar by weight	Restrictions on beverages sold in vending machines	Restrictions on access to vending machines	Notes
Yes. State policy prohibits an elementary school campus from serving competitive foods or FMNV to students anywhere on school premises until the end of the last scheduled class (does not pertain to food items made available by the school food service program).	An elementary school may not serve or provide access to FMNV, all other forms of candy, or competitive foods at any time, anywhere on school premises until the end of the last scheduled class.	An elementary school may not serve or provide access to FMNV, all other forms of candy, or competitive foods at any time, anywhere on school premises until the end of the last scheduled class.	An elementary school may not serve or provide access to FMNV, all other forms of candy or competitive foods at any time, anywhere on school premises until the end of the last scheduled class.	Portion size restrictions are placed on certain food and beverage items served or made available to students, with the exception of school meals. State policy places restrictions on portion size for the following items: chips, baked chips, crackers, popcorn, cereal, trail mix, nuts, seeds, dried fruit, jerky, pretzels, cookies/cereal bars, bakery items, frozen desserts, yogurt, ice cream, pudding, gelatin, and beverage items. Elementary classrooms may allow one nutritious snack per day, but not at the same time as the regular meal period for that class. The snack must comply with the fat and sugar limits of the Public School Nutrition Policy and may not contain any FMNVs or consist of candy or dessert type items.

continued

Additional restrictions on vending machine

TABLE C-1 Continued

		Nutrition standards for competitive foods sold in schools (includes items sold à la carte, in school stores and/or vending machines)			
State	Grade Level	Does the state have nutritional standards for competitive foods?	Max. calories from fat	Max. calories from saturated fat	Max. % of sugar by weight
Texas (cont.)	Middle (Grades 6, 7, 8)/Junior High (Grades 7 and 8 or Grades 7, 8 and 9)	Yes	Schools and other vendors may not serve food items containing more than 28 g of fat per serving size more than twice per week. By the 2006-07 school year, the goal is to reduce this to 23 g of fat. French fries and other fried potato products must not exceed 3 oz per serving, may not be offered more than three times per week, and students may only purchase one serving at a time. Schools serving potato chips should use reduced fat, no more than 5 g per oz, or baked varieties when possible.	Not specified	Flavored or unflavored milks and other beverages may contain no more than 30 g total sugar per 8 oz serving. Frozen fruit slushes must contain a minimum of 50% fruit juice.

	Additional restrictions on vending machine			
Additional restrictions	Max. calories from fat, saturated fat, and sugar by weight	Restrictions on beverages sold in vending machines	Restrictions on access to vending machines	Notes
Yes. Prohibits a middle or junior high school from serving or providing access to FMNV and all other forms of candy at any time, anywhere on school premises until after the last lunch period. Competitive foods may not be served to students anywhere on school campus during school meals. Beginning in 2006-07 school year, schools should reduce the purchase of any products containing trans fats. Schools also must abide by maximum portion sizes outlined in the Texas Public School Nutrition Policy.	Must meet nutrition standards as previously described.	Prohibits a middle or junior high school from serving or providing access to FMNV and all other forms of candy at any time, anywhere on school premises until after the last lunch period. Competitive foods may not be served to students anywhere on school campus during school meals.	Prohibits a middle or junior high school from serving or providing access to FMNV and all other forms of candy at any time, anywhere on school premises until after the last lunch period. Competitive foods may not be served to students anywhere on school campus during school meals.	Portion size restrictions are placed on certain food and beverage items served or made available to students, with the exception of school meals. State policy places restrictions on portion size for the following items: chips, baked chips, crackers, popcorn, cereal, trail mix, nuts, seeds, dried fruit, jerky, pretzels, cookies/cereal bars, bakery items, frozen desserts, ice cream, pudding, gelatin, yogurt, candy bar and packaged candies, frozen fruit slushes and beverage items.

continued

TABLE C-1 Continued

State	Grade Level	Nutrition standards for competitive foods sold in schools (includes items sold à la carte, in school stores and/or vending machines)			
		Does the state have nutritional standards for competitive foods?	Max. calories from fat	Max. calories from saturated fat	Max. % of sugar by weight
Texas (cont.)	High School	Yes	Schools and other vendors may not serve food items containing more than 28 g of fat per serving size more than twice per week. By the 2006-2007 school year, the goal is to reduce this to 23 g of fat. French fries and other fried potato products must not exceed 3 oz per serving, may not be offered more than three times per week, and student may only purchase one serving at a time.	Not specified	Flavored or unflavored milks and other beverages, including those restricted as FMNV, may not contain more than 30 g total sugar per 8 oz serving. Frozen fruit slushes must contain a minimum of 50% fruit juice.
Utah	Elementary, Middle, and High Schools	No	N/A	N/A	N/A

| | Additional restrictions on vending machine | | | |
| | Max. calories from fat, saturated fat, and sugar by weight | Restrictions on beverages sold in vending machines | Restrictions on access to vending machines | Notes |
Additional restrictions				
No. Does not allow sale of FMNVs or competitive foods in food service areas where federal school meals are served. Beginning in 2006-07 school year, schools should reduce the purchase of any products containing trans fats. Schools also must abide by maximum portion sizes outlined in the Texas Public School Nutrition Policy.	Must meet nutrition standards as previously described.	Prohibits the sale of sugared, carbonated beverages in containers larger than 12 oz. Does not allow sale of FMNVs or competitive foods in food service areas where federal school meals are served.	Does not allow sale of FMNVs or competitive foods in food service areas where federal school meals are served.	Portion size restrictions are placed on certain food and beverage items served or made available to students, with the exception of school meals. State policy places restrictions on portion size for the following items: chips, baked chips, crackers, popcorn, cereal, trail mix, nuts, seeds, dried fruit, jerky, pretzels, cookies/cereal bars, bakery items, frozen desserts, ice cream, pudding, gelatin, yogurt, candy bar and packaged candies, frozen fruit slushes and beverage items. Portion sizes for high school students in comparison to elementary and middle school students are larger.
No	N/A	None	None	None

continued

TABLE C-1 Continued

| State | Grade Level | Nutrition standards for competitive foods sold in schools (includes items sold à la carte, in school stores and/or vending machines) | | | |
		Does the state have nutritional standards for competitive foods?	Max. calories from fat	Max. calories from saturated fat	Max. % of sugar by weight
Vermont	Elementary, Middle, and High Schools	No	N/A	N/A	N/A
Virginia	Elementary, Middle, and High Schools	No	N/A	N/A	N/A

| Additional restrictions | Additional restrictions on vending machine | | | Notes |
	Max. calories from fat, saturated fat, and sugar by weight	Restrictions on beverages sold in vending machines	Restrictions on access to vending machines	
No	N/A	None	None	During 2004 session, H.B. 272 was enacted requiring the Department of Education to develop a model school fitness and nutrition policy, which includes a definition of nutritious foods, nutritional guidelines regarding foods sold or served by the food service program, vending machines, snack bars and school stores. Schools are not required to adopt model policy.
The sale of food items for the profit of any entity other than the school nutrition program is prohibited during the lunch period and from 6:00 am through the end of the last breakfast service.	N/A	None	The sale of food items for the profit of any entity other than the school nutrition program is prohibited during the lunch period and from 6:00 am through the end of the last breakfast service.	None

continued

TABLE C-1 Continued

State	Grade Level	Nutrition standards for competitive foods sold in schools (includes items sold à la carte, in school stores and/or vending machines)			
		Does the state have nutritional standards for competitive foods?	Max. calories from fat	Max. calories from saturated fat	Max. % of sugar by weight
Washington	Elementary, Middle, and High Schools	No	N/A	N/A	N/A
West Virginia	Elementary, Middle, and High Schools	Yes	Limited to not more than 8 g of fat per one oz serving or meet USDA standards for a lunch component.	Not specified	40%
Wisconsin	Elementary, Middle, and High Schools	No	N/A	N/A	N/A

| Additional restrictions | Additional restrictions on vending machine | | | |
	Max. calories from fat, saturated fat, and sugar by weight	Restrictions on beverages sold in vending machines	Restrictions on access to vending machines	Notes
No	N/A	None	None	Legislation enacted in 2004 requires Washington State School Directors Association to develop model school nutrition policy but does not require schools to adopt the policy. Schools are required to have a policy.
No candy, soft drinks (exception for high school), chewing gum or flavored ice bars will be sold or served during the school day. All "other foods" will reflect the Dietary Guidelines or meet the USDA standard for a lunch component (see notes for definition of "other foods"). Only meal components may be sold as à la carte items for breakfast, and only fluid milk, milk shakes and bottled water may be sold as à la carte items for lunch. Any juice or juice product sold or served must contain a minimum of 20% fruit juice.	All "other foods" made available will follow the nutritional guidelines as indicated.	Soft drinks may not be sold in elementary, middle or junior high schools through vending machines, in school stores or on-site fund-raisers during the school day. Schools are only permitted to sell "healthy beverages" during the school day, defined as water, 100% fruit and vegetable juice, low-fat milk and other juice beverages with at least 20% real juice. For those high schools that permit the sale of soft drinks, "healthy beverages" must account for at least 50% of the total beverages offered and must be located near the vending machines containing soft drinks.	No candy, soft drinks (exception for high schools), chewing gum, or flavored ice bars will be sold or served during the school day.	"Other foods" are defined as any food or beverage, other than those served as part of the school meal, including snacks from vending machines, foods sold during school hours for fund-raising, and foods served at parties. "Other foods" do not include those brought to school by individual students for their own consumption.
No	N/A	None	None	None

continued

TABLE C-1 Continued

| State | Grade Level | Nutrition standards for competitive foods sold in schools (includes items sold à la carte, in school stores and/or vending machines) | | | |
		Does the state have nutritional standards for competitive foods?	Max. calories from fat	Max. calories from saturated fat	Max. % of sugar by weight
Wyoming	Elementary, Middle, and High Schools	No	N/A	N/A	N/A

*The regulations for the Federal School Lunch Program and the School Breakfast Program do not prohibit the sale of foods in competition with reimbursable meals as long as those foods are not considered to be foods of minimal nutritional value. These FMNV may not be sold or served in food service areas during breakfast or lunch. Exceptions to the rule are specified by the USDA.

*The USDA categorizes foods of minimal nutritional value as soda water (which includes carbonated beverages), water ices (except those that contain fruit or fruit juices), chewing gum, and certain candies (including hard candy, jellies and gums, marshmallow candies, fondant, licorice, spun candy and candy-coated popcorn).

SOURCE: Health Policy Tracking Service, a service of Thomson West. Data current as of December 31, 2005.

| | Additional restrictions on vending machine | | | |
Additional restrictions	Max. calories from fat, saturated fat, and sugar by weight	Restrictions on beverages sold in vending machines	Restrictions on access to vending machines	Notes
No	N/A	None	None	School districts can make their policies stricter.

Guidelines for Competitive Foods and Beverages

The Alliance for a Healthier Generation was formed by the American Heart Association and the William J. Clinton Foundation. A product of the Alliance, the Nutrition Guidelines for Competitive Foods for K-12, developed out of a collaboration between the Alliance and the Campbell Soup Company, Dannon, Kraft Foods, Mars, Inc., and PepsiCo. The guidelines were developed in conjunction with nutrition experts at the American Heart Association to provide science-based and age-appropriate information to help children in schools make healthier food choices. The criteria established by the guidelines are designed to promote nutrient-rich foods, fat-free and low-fat dairy products, and place limits on calories, fat, saturated fat, trans fat, sugar, and sodium.

Guidelines for Competitive Foods Sold in Schools to Students[1]

These guidelines apply to snacks, side items, treats, and desserts offered for sale as Competitive Foods in schools. All such Competitive Foods shall meet one of the following numbered criteria.

These foods include but are not limited to fruits, vegetables, yogurts (including drinkable yogurt and yogurt smoothies), puddings, soups, cheeses, snack chips (e.g., potato, tortilla, corn, veggie, etc.), pretzels, crackers,

---

[1]Alliance for a Healthier Generation, a program of the Clinton Foundation; Website: www.HealthierGeneration.org.

popcorn, nuts, seeds, french fries, dried meat snacks, granola bars, energy bars, breakfast bars, health bars, cookies, brownies, snack cakes, coffee cakes, pastries, doughnuts, danishes, candy, confectionery, chocolate, ice cream, frozen yogurt, sherbet, ice pops, frozen fruit bars, and other similar foods.

Items that would be considered to be entrées if sold in the reimbursable meal program, but are sold à la carte as Competitive Foods, are not subject to these Guidelines.

1. Any fruit with no added sweeteners or vegetables that are non-fried. Since fresh fruits and vegetables vary in size and calories naturally, they have no calorie limit. However, calories for packaged fruits and vegetables are easily ascertained according to package nutrition labeling. As such, calorie limits for these fruits and vegetables are specified as follows:

	Elementary	Middle	High
fresh	no limit	no limit	no limit
packaged in own juice	150	180	200
dried	150	180	200

2. Any reduced-fat or part-skim cheese ≤ 1.5 oz.
3. Any one egg with no added fat or equal amount of egg equivalent with no added fat.
4. Any other food that meets all of the following criteria:
    a. ≤ 35% of total calories from fat
        i.   Nuts, nut butters, and seeds are exempt from above limitation and are permitted.
        ii. Products described in Addendum 1 are exempt and are permitted until August 31, 2008.
    b. ≤ 10% of calories from saturated fat -OR- ≤ 1g saturated fat
    c. 0 g trans fat
    d. ≤ 35% sugar by weight
    e. ≤ 230 mg sodium
        i.   Lowfat and fat-free dairy products can have ≤ 480mg sodium.
        ii. Vegetables with sauce, and soups can have ≤ 480mg sodium if they contain one or more of the following: ≥ 2g fiber; or ≥ 5g protein; or ≥ 10% DV of Vitamin A, C, E, folate, calcium, magnesium, potassium, or iron; or ≥ 1/2 serving (1/4 cup) of fruit or vegetables.
        iii. Soups described in Addendum 2 are exempt and are permitted until August 31, 2008.

f. If products are dairy, they must be non-fat or low fat dairy.
g. Meet 1 of the following calorie requirements:
    i.   ≤ 100 calories
    ii. Vegetables with sauce and soups meeting 4.e above can
         have 150 calories if they contain two or more of the fol-
         lowing: ≥ 2g fiber; or ≥ 5g protein; or ≥ 10% DV of Vi-
         tamin A, C, E, folate, calcium, magnesium, potassium, or
         iron; or ≥ 1/2 serving (1/4 cup) of fruit or vegetables.
    iii. Other foods can have calorie limits per below if they con-
         tain one or more of the following: ≥ 2g fiber; or ≥ 5g
         protein; or ≥ 10% DV of Vitamin A, C, E, folate, calcium,
         magnesium, potassium, or iron; or ≥ 1/2 serving (1/4 cup)
         of fruit or vegetables:
         • ≤ 150 calories for elementary schools
         • ≤ 180 calories for middle school
         • ≤ 200 calories for high school.

For individual serving packages, these nutritional Guidelines are defined
for a whole package as labeled on the package's Nutrition Facts panel. In
the event that the food is bought in bulk but served individually, such as
on an à la carte line, then the criteria apply to the serving size actually offered to students.

Time of Day

These Guidelines shall apply to items sold on school grounds or at school
activities during the regular and extended school day when events are
primarily under the control of the school or third parties on behalf of the
school. The extended school day is defined as the time before or after the
official school day that includes activities such as clubs, yearbook, band
and choir practice, student government, drama, sports practices, intramural
sports, and childcare/latchkey programs. These Guidelines shall also apply
to food supplied by schools during official transportation to and from
school and school sponsored activities, including but not limited to field
trips and interscholastic sporting events where the school is the visiting
team except as specified herein.

These Guidelines do not apply to school sponsored or school related bona
fide fundraising activities that take place off school grounds and not in
transit to and from school. Nor do they apply to booster sales at school
related events where parents and other adults are a significant part of
an audience or are selling food as boosters either during intermission
or immediately before or after such events. These school related events
frequently occur during evenings and weekends. Examples of these events

include but are not limited to interscholastic sporting events, school plays, and band concerts.

Addendum 1—Total and Saturated Fats

The American Heart Association Dietary and Lifestyle Recommendations released June 2006 emphasized saturated fat—setting lower goals for the amount of saturated fat in the diet. Given that the Recommendations encourage people to consume ≤ 7% of calories from saturated fat while meeting total fat recommendations of ≤ 35% and with the intent of encouraging food manufacturers to develop products to meet this goal, products with ≤ 7% of calories from saturated fat will be allowed to have ≤ 40% of calories from total fat until August 31, 2008. This transition period will provide manufacturers time to reformulate these products such that they provide ≤ 35% of calories from total fat by August 31, 2008.

Addendum 2—Sodium

A variety of commercially available soup products available in bulk through food service channels to schools can meet all the requirements specified in the Guidelines except for an upper limit of 480 mg for sodium. In recognition of this market availability, soups that meet the sodium requirement specified in this Addendum will be considered to meet the Guidelines until August 31, 2008. This transition period will provide manufacturers time for product reformulation, as well as the ability to meet manufacturing and food service distribution requirements.

Soups with ≤ 750 mg sodium are permitted if they contain one or more of the following: ≥ 2g fiber; or ≥ 5g protein; or ≥ 10% DV of Vitamin A, C, E, folate, calcium, magnesium, potassium, or iron; or ≥ 1/2 serving (1/4 cup) of fruit or vegetables.

Guidelines for Beverages Sold in Schools to Students[2]

Helping schools provide healthy settings for their students is a top priority for the Alliance for a Healthier Generation. These School Beverage Guidelines were developed to serve as the beverage criteria for the Healthy Schools Program. They will accelerate the shift to lower-calorie and nutritious beverages that children consume during the regular and extended school day. These Guidelines have been adopted by the American Beverage Association, PepsiCo, Coca-Cola and Cadbury Schweppes as their school beverage policy.

---

[2]Alliance for a Healthier Generation, a program of the Clinton Foundation; Website: (www. HealthierGeneration.org).

Elementary School
- Water
- Up to 8 ounce servings of milk and 100% juice
  - o Fat-free or low fat regular and flavored milk with up to 150 calories/8 ounces*
  - o 100% juice with no added sweeteners, up to 120 calories/8 ounces, and with at least 10% of the recommended daily value for three or more vitamins and minerals

Middle School
- Water
- Up to 10 ounce servings of milk and 100% juice
  - o Fat-free or low fat regular or flavored milk with up to 150 calories/8 ounces*
  - o 100% juice with no added sweeteners, up to 120 calories/8 ounces, and with at least 10% of the recommended daily value for three or more vitamins and minerals
- As a practical matter, if middle school and high school students have shared access to areas on a common campus or in common buildings, then the school community has the option to adopt the high school standard.

High School
- Water
- No or low calorie beverages with up to 10 calories/8 ounces
- Up to 12 ounce servings of milk, 100% juice, and certain other drinks
  - o Fat-free or low fat regular and flavored milk with up to 150 calories/8 ounces*
  - o 100% juice with no added sweeteners, up to 120 calories/8 ounces, and with at least 10% of the recommended daily value for three or more vitamins and minerals
  - o Other drinks with no more than 66 calories/8 ounces
- At least 50% of non-milk beverages must be water and no- or low-calorie options

The Guidelines apply to all beverages (outside of the school meal) sold to students on school grounds during the regular and extended school day. The extended school day includes before and after school activities like clubs, yearbook, band, student government, drama and childcare/latchkey programs.

These School Beverage Guidelines do not apply to school-related events (such as interscholastic sporting events, school plays, and band concerts) where parents and other adults constitute a significant portion of the audience or are selling beverages as boosters.

Milk includes nutritionally equivalent milk alternatives per USDA. In recognition of the currently limited availability of flavored milk with less than 150 calories/8 oz and the importance of milk's natural nutrients in children's diets, flavored milk with up to 180 calories/8 oz will be allowed under these guidelines until August 31, 2008 so long as schools attempt to buy the lowest calorie flavored milk available to them. Because of unique CA state milk regulations, the calorie limit for fat-free and low fat flavored milk in CA schools is 180 calories/8 oz with a transition period until August 31, 2008 that allows 210 calories/8 oz.

APPENDIX
E

Open Sessions

NUTRITION STANDARDS FOR FOODS IN SCHOOLS

October 26, 2005
The National Academy of Sciences Building
2100 C Street, NW
Washington, DC

Background, Perspectives on Project, and Discussion
Moderated by Virginia Stallings, Committee Chair:
- Derek Miller, Professional Staff, U.S. Senate, Committee on Agriculture, Nutrition, and Forestry
- Shirley Watkins, Member, IOM Committee on Prevention of Obesity in Children and Youth
- Linda Meyers, Director, Food and Nutrition Board, Institute of Medicine, National Academies
- Jay Hirschman, Director, Special Nutrition Staff, Office of Analysis, Nutrition and Evaluation, Food and Nutrition Service, U.S. Department of Agriculture
- Mary McKenna, Sponsor Representative, Division of Adolescent and School Health, Centers for Disease Control and Prevention

PERSPECTIVES ON NUTRITION STANDARDS
FOR FOODS IN SCHOOLS

December 5, 2005
The National Academy of Sciences Building
2100 C Street, NW
Washington, DC

Panel Discussion by Invited Speakers
Moderated by Virginia Stallings, Committee Chair:
- Karen Weber Cullen, Ph.D., R.D., L.D., Associate Professor of Pediatrics-Behavioral Nutrition, Baylor College of Medicine, Houston, TX
- Barbara O. Schneeman, Ph.D., Director, Office of Nutritional Products, Labeling and Dietary Supplements, Center for Food Safety and Applied Nutrition, Food and Drug Administration College Park, MD
- Margo Wootan, D.Sc., Director of Nutrition Policy, Center for Science in the Public Interest, Washington, DC
- Alicia Moag-Stahlberg, M.S., R.D., L.D., Executive Director, Action for Healthy Kids
- Susan Neely, C.E.O. and President, American Beverage Association

Panel Discussion with Representatives of the Food Industry
Moderated by Karen Cullen, Ph.D., R.D., L.D., Associate Professor of Pediatrics-Behavioral Nutrition, Baylor College of Medicine, Houston, TX:
- Nancy Green, Ph.D., Vice President, Health and Wellness, Pepsi Beverages and Foods, PepsiCo
- Melanie White, Director, Education and Youth Channels, Coca-Cola North America
- Richard Black, Ph.D., Vice-President, Global Nutrition, Kraft Foods, Inc.
- Kathy Wiemer, M.S., R.D., L.D., Senior Manager, General Mills Bell Institute of Health and Nutrition
- Hope Hale, M.S., R.D., C.D., Principal Nutrition Scientist, Schwan Food Company
- Susan Waltman, B.S., Vice President of Nutrition, ConAgra Foods, Inc.

Public Comments
Moderated by Virginia Stallings, Committee Chair:
* Barbara Dennison, M.D., American Heart Association
* Dulcie Ward, Physician's Committee for Responsible Medicine
* Robert Earl, Food Products Association
* Michelle Matto, International Dairy Foods Association
* Keith Ayoob, Ed.D., R.D., FADA., Department of Pediatrics, Albert Einstein College of Medicine
* Susan Rubin, Westchester Coalition for Better School Food
* Helen Phillips, Nutrition Committee Chair, School Nutrition Association
* Robert Schwartz, M.D., American Academy of Pediatrics
* Martine Brizius, National Association of State Boards of Education
* Jill Nicholls, National Dairy Council
* Barbara A. Nabrit-Stephens, M.D., National Medical Association
* Jennifer MacAulay, Senior Manager of Scientific and Nutrition Policy, Grocery Manufacturers Association
* Dr. Rebecca Reeves, President, American Dietetic Association
* Jacqueline R. Berning, Ph.D., R.D., Associate Professor, University of Colorado, Colorado Springs

EXPERIENCE IN DEVELOPMENT, IMPLEMENTATION, AND EVALUATION OF NUTRITION STANDARDS IN SCHOOLS

February 13, 2006
Arnold and Mabel Beckman Center of the National Academies
100 Academy Drive
Irvine, CA

Discussion by Invited Speakers
Moderated by Virginia Stallings, Committee Chair:
* Harold Goldstein, Dr.P.H., Executive Director, California Center for Public Health Advocacy, Davis
* Marilyn Wells, M.A., R.D., Director of Food Service, Los Angeles Unified School District
* Gail Woodward-Lopez, M.P.H., R.D., Associate Director, Center for Weight and Health, University of California, Berkeley
* Mary Kay Harrison, M.S., formerly Executive Director, West Virginia Department of Education, Charleston

- Jonathan D. Shenkin, D.D.S., M.P.H., Penobscot Children's Dentistry Associates, Bangor, ME; Assistant Clinical Professor of Health Policy, Goldman School of Dental Medicine, Boston University
- John Perkins, Senior Policy Advisor for Food and Nutrition, Texas Department of Agriculture, Austin
- Michael Rosenberger, Food Service Director, Irving Independent School District, Texas

LESSONS LEARNED FROM DEVELOPMENT OF FEDERAL NUTRITION STANDARDS FOR THE SCHOOL MEAL PROGRAMS

April 21, 2006
The Keck Center of the National Academies
500 Fifth Street, NW
Washington, DC

Discussion by Invited Speakers
Moderated by Virginia Stallings, Committee Chair: Presentations from the Child Nutrition Division, Food and Nutrition Service, U.S Department of Agriculture
- Stanley Garnet, Director
- Robert (Bob) Eadie, Chief, Policy and Program Development Branch
- Clare Miller, M.S., R.D., Senior Nutritionist

APPENDIX
F

Committee Member
Biographical Sketches

VIRGINIA A. STALLINGS, M.D. (*Chair*), is the Jean A. Cortner Endowed Chair in Pediatric Gastroenterology, Director of the Nutrition Center, and Director of Faculty Development at the Joseph Stokes Jr. Research Institute at the Children's Hospital of Philadelphia. Dr. Stallings is also a Professor of Pediatrics at the University of Pennsylvania School of Medicine. Her pediatric nutrition research interests include evaluation of dietary intake and energy expenditure, and nutrition-related chronic disease. Her current research is funded by the National Institutes of Health and foundations. Dr. Stallings served on numerous IOM projects including the Committee on Nutrition Services for Medicare Beneficiaries (Chair), Committee on the Scientific Basis for Dietary Risk Eligibility Criteria for WIC Programs (Chair), Committee to Review the WIC Food Packages (member), and the Food and Nutrition Board (Co-Vice Chair). Dr. Stallings earned a B.S. degree in nutrition and foods from Auburn University, an M.S. degree in human nutrition and biochemistry from Cornell University, and an M.D. degree from the School of Medicine of the University of Alabama in Birmingham. She completed a pediatric residency at the University of Virginia and a pediatric nutrition fellowship at the Hospital for Sick Children, Toronto, Ontario. Dr. Stallings is board certified in pediatrics and clinical nutrition, and a member of the Institute of Medicine.

DENNIS M. BIER, M.D., is Professor of Pediatrics and Director of the USDA/ARS Children's Nutrition Research Center at the Baylor College of Medicine, Houston, Texas. His research interests include hormonal regulation of metabolic fuel transport; human nutrition, growth, and development; maternal-fetal nutrition; and the nutritional developmental origins of adult chronic disease. Dr. Bier served as Co-President of the American Society for Nutrition, as President of the International Pediatric Research Foundation, as a member of the FDA Food Advisory Committee, and as a member of the 1995 USDA/HHS Dietary Guidelines Advisory Committee. He served on the IOM Food and Nutrition Board as well as IOM and National Research Council projects including the Committee for Prevention of Obesity in Children and Youth, Committee on Dioxins and Dioxin-like Compounds in the Food Supply, Committee on Adolescent Health and Development, and Workshop on the Synthesis of Research on Adolescent Health and Development. Dr. Bier currently serves as Chair of the Food and Nutrition Board, Chairman of the Board of the International Life Sciences Institute (ILSI) Research Foundation, member of the ILSI Board of Trustees, and member of the FDA Pediatric Advisory Committee. Dr. Bier serves on the Expert Advisory Panel on Nutrition and Electrolytes of the U.S. Pharmacopeial Convention, Inc.; the Mars Nutrition Research Council; and the McDonald's Global Advisory Council on Balanced, Active Lifestyles. He has also served as consultant for other food industry organizations including the Sugar Association and the Corn Refiners Association. Dr. Bier earned a B.S. degree from Le Moyne College and an M.D. degree from New Jersey College of Medicine. He is board certified in pediatrics and is a member of the Institute of Medicine.

MARGIE TUDOR BRADFORD, R.N., is a member of the School Board of Bardstown Independent School District in Kentucky (1979–2006). She is a former member and past President of the Kentucky School Boards Association (KSBA) Board of Directors and has served on numerous local, state, and national committees engaged in school health issues. Ms. Bradford is a former member of the National School Boards Association (NSBA) Board of Directors (1996-2002), a peer-elected position. Ms. Bradford served as chairman of the School Health Advisory Committee for that period of time, on an advisory steering committee on state and local school policies and programs on physical activity, healthy eating, and tobacco use prevention (NSBA/National Association of State Boards of Education). She also served on the National Coordinating Committee on School Health and the central steering committee to develop guidelines for school health programs (American Academy of Pediatrics/National Association of School Nurses). She was honored as a Healthy School Hero at the 2002 Healthy Schools Summit. Ms. Bradford is a Registered Nurse and focuses her advocacy activities on health and wellness of students, including serving on the Kentucky Child Now! Board of Directors. She also reports to the KSBA Board of Directors on coordinated school health issues efforts in Kentucky.

CARLOS A. CAMARGO, JR., M.D., DR.P.H., is an Associate Professor of Medicine and Epidemiology at Harvard Medical School, and an Associate Physician at both the Massachusetts General Hospital and Brigham & Women's Hospital in Boston. His epidemiology research has focused on the relation of diet, exercise, and obesity on risk of developing asthma. He is a past president of the American College of Epidemiology and serves as a member of several national committees concerned with diverse topics in clinical medicine and public health. For example, Dr. Camargo served on the 2005 U.S. Dietary Guidelines Advisory Committee and on the National Asthma Education and Prevention Program's Third Expert Panel (the group that wrote the national asthma guidelines). He has more than 220 peer-reviewed publications. Dr. Camargo earned a B.A. degree in human biology from Stanford University, an M.P.H. degree from the University of California–Berkeley, an M.D. degree from the University of California–San Francisco, and a Dr.P.H. degree from the Harvard School of Public Health.

ISOBEL R. CONTENTO, PH.D., is the Mary Rose Professor of Nutrition and Education and Coordinator of the Program in Nutrition, Department of Health and Behavior Studies, at Teachers College, Columbia University, New York. Her research expertise is in behavioral aspects of nutrition; use of psychosocial theory to study factors influencing food choice and decision-making processes, particularly among children and adolescents; children's and adolescents' understandings of the impact of food and food systems on the environment; and development and evaluation of nutrition education curricula and programs. Dr. Contento is co-developer of Linking Food and the Environment (LiFE), an inquiry-based curriculum which helps teach urban children about how foods are preserved, packaged, and processed, and the resulting impact on the environment. She is currently conducting a study on childhood overweight prevention in middle school students through a science education-based program called Choice, Control and Change. She served on advisory committees for the American Cancer Society, the Centers for Disease Control and Prevention, and the U.S. Department of Agriculture. Dr. Contento earned a B.S. degree from the University of Edinburgh, UK, and a Ph.D. degree from the University of California–Berkeley.

THOMAS H. COOK, PH.D., R.N., F.N.P., is an Assistant Professor of Nursing at Vanderbilt University's School of Nursing, Nashville, Tennessee. His research interests include health policy development, program evaluation, and the prevention of cardiovascular disease through the use of nutrition and physical education programs in children. Dr. Cook is also a School Health Researcher for Monroe Carell Jr. Children's Hospital at Vanderbilt.

In this role, he is heading a partnership with Children's Hospital and the Metro Nashville Public Schools (nearly 72,000 students in 129 schools) to provide health assessments using the Centers for Disease Control's nine component model for a healthy school. He earned a B.S.N. degree from Loyola University, an F.N.P. degree from Albany Medical College/Russell Sage College, an M.S.N. degree in cardiovascular nursing from St. Louis University, and a Ph.D. degree from Vanderbilt University. Dr. Cook is a Registered Nurse and a Family Nurse Practitioner.

ERIC A. DECKER, PH.D., is a Professor in the Department of Food Science at the University of Massachusetts–Amherst, and holds the Fergus Clydesdale Endowed Chair. Dr. Decker's research interests are in food chemistry and include methods to increase the bioavailability and prevent the oxidative deterioration of lipids linked to progression of diseases such as cardiovascular disease. He serves in various professional organizations such as the Institute of Food Technologists (IFT; Chair of the Food Chemistry Division) and the American Meat Science Association (Board of Directors). Dr. Decker's honors include Malcolm Trout Visiting Scholar, Michigan State University; Visiting Scientist, Linus Pauling Institute, Oregon State University; Guest Professor, Huazhong Agricultural University, China; Samuel Cate Prescott Award, IFT; Hokkaido Overseas Guest Researcher Fellowship, Hokkaido Food Processing Research Center, Japan; and Future Leader Award, ILSI. He was coeditor of Current Protocols in Food Analytical Chemistry, 2002. Dr. Decker earned a B.S. degree in biology from Pennsylvania State University, an M.S. degree in food science and nutrition from Washington State University, and a Ph.D. in food science and nutrition from the University of Massachusetts–Amherst.

ROSEMARY DEDERICHS, B.A., is the Director of the Food Services Department for the Minneapolis Public School District, Minnesota. She has worked with the school district for 20 years, serving as a Food Service Assistant, Site Manager, Multisite Coordinator, Operations Manager, Interim Director, and currently as Director. Ms. Dederichs' began her career in schools as a certified elementary school teacher. At present she is certified as a State and City Food Manager and certified at Level III in Child Nutrition through the National School Nutrition Association. Ms. Dederichs is a former executive board member of the Minnesota School Nutrition Association and served on the Gold Medal Advisory Board for General Mills, Inc. She received the Golden Apple Award for Nutrition Education from the Minnesota Food Service Association and a Community Partner Star Award from the University of Minnesota School of Public Health, Environmental Health Sciences Division, in recognition of her contributions to the guidance of Minneapolis Public Schools students. She was also a corecipient of the Allina Health Systems 2006 Healthy Community Award for developing healthier menus for her students. Ms. Dederichs earned a B.A. degree in psychology from Mundelein College of Loyola University and conducted additional studies in education at Northern Illinois University, College of DuPage, and Elmhurst College.

JAY T. ENGELN, M.ED., is a Resident Practitioner in School/Business Partnerships with the National Association of Secondary School Principals (NASSP), Reston, Virginia. Mr. Engeln held positions in secondary education as a teacher of biology, environmental science, anatomy and physiology, and coach of soccer and hockey. He served as Assistant Principal (Coronado High School, Colorado Springs, Colorado) and Principal (William J. Palmer High School, Colorado Springs, CO; Mountain Vista High School, Highlands Ranch, CO). Mr. Engeln's honors include the Evanston Township High School Stuart Merrell Memorial Award for Citizenship and Service to Youth (1980), Colorado Soccer Coach of the Year (1982, 1984), National High School Soccer Coach of the Year (1985, National Coach Magazine), U.S. West Outstanding Teacher Award (1989), Colorado College Education Department–Kappa Delta Pi Award for outstanding contributions to education (1998), Colorado Association of Executives–Colorado Principal of the Year (1999), National Association of Secondary School Principals–National Principal of the Year (2000), Business Advisory Council–Honorary Colorado State Chairman (2004), and Colorado Businessperson of the Year (2004, National Republican Congressional Committee). Mr. Engeln's current position is one of several Resident Practitioner positions at NASSP supported by external funding. Mr. Engeln's position, the Resident Practitioner in School/Business Partnerships, is currently supported by a grant from the Coca-Cola Company. Mr. Engeln earned a B.A. degree in biology from Colorado College and an M.Ed. degree in science from the University of Colorado. His studies continued at the University of Denver, and he holds Secondary School Administration Certification. Mr. Engeln received a Doctor of Science, honoris causa, from Colorado College. He currently resides in Colorado.

BARBARA N. FISH, M.A., is immediate Past President of the West Virginia Board of Education, a former classroom teacher, and a long-time community volunteer and child advocate. She currently chairs the State Board of Education's Wellness Committee. While Mrs. Fish served as President, the Board approved Standards for School Nutrition, establishing statewide standards for foods and beverages sold to students in schools. She also serves as Secretary of the State's School Building Authority, member of the West Virginia Commission for Professional Teaching Standards, in addition to other education boards and commissions. Prior to her appointment to the State Board of Education, she served on the Commission for National and Community Service, also a gubernatorial appointment. Mrs. Fish has assumed major leadership roles in numerous school and community organizations. She earned a B.A. degree in Spanish from Grove City College, an M.A. degree in Spanish from West Chester State College with additional study at the Universidad de Salamanca. Mrs. Fish is a former Spanish language teacher and received honorary induction into Delta Kappa Gamma Society International, a professional honorary society of women educators. She has received several awards for volunteerism and advocacy of children's issues.

TRACY A. FOX, M.P.H., R.D., L.D., is a Nutrition Consultant and the President of Food, Nutrition, and Policy Consultants, LLC. Previously, Ms. Fox held positions as Senior Federal Regulatory Manager with the American Dietetic Association, Division of Government Relations, Washington, DC; Food Program Specialist in the Child Nutrition Division and Assistant to the Associate Administrator with the U.S. Department of Agriculture, Food and Nutrition Service, Alexandria, Virginia; Manager of Federal Systems Division with Maximus, Inc., Falls Church, Virginia; Instructor of Food Preparation and Meal Management at Hood College, Frederick, Maryland; and dietitian in food management and clinical dietetics with the U.S. Navy. Ms. Fox has experience in the formulation of nutrition standards for federally reimbursable school meals at the federal level and formulation of nutrition standards for non-reimbursable foods in schools at state and local levels. Ms. Fox serves on various school health boards and committees at the federal, state, and local levels. She represents the Society for Nutrition Education on the Action for Healthy Kids Partner Steering Committee, is on the board of the Maryland Healthy Schools Coalition, Co-Chairs the Montgomery County School Health Council and Chairs the Health Committee of the Montgomery County Council of Parent-Teacher Associations. Ms. Fox earned a B.S. degree through the coordinated undergraduate program in dietetics at Hood College and an M.P.H. degree at the Graduate School of Public Health of University of Pittsburgh. She is a Registered Dietitian with licensure. Ms. Fox currently resides in Bethesda, MD.

JAMES C. OHLS, PH.D., is a consultant on low-income policy issues. His former position was with Mathematica Policy Research (MPR), Inc., Princeton, New Jersey, where he was a Senior Fellow and Area Leader for Food and Nutrition Policy. Before joining MPR, Dr. Ohls was an Assistant Professor of Economics and Public Affairs at Princeton University, Princeton. Dr. Ohls research interests include the evaluation of nutrition programs, how policies and changes in policies affect nutrition programs, how nutrition programs operate administratively (including their efficiency

and effectiveness), and how nutrition programs reach the target populations. He has 20 years of experience in designing and conducting program
and policy evaluations and has conducted numerous studies of the food
stamp and school nutrition programs. Dr. Ohls is co-author of the book
The Food Stamp Program: Design Tradeoffs, Policy, and Impacts (1993)
and the report Reaching More Hungry Children: The Seamless Summer
Food Waiver (2003). Additional research on children includes a study on
home resources and children's achievement (1981). Dr. Ohls earned a B.A.
degree in economics from Harvard College and a Ph.D. degree in economics
from the University of Pennsylvania.

LYNN PARKER, M.S., is the director of Child Nutrition Programs and Nutrition Policy at the Food Research and Action Center (FRAC), a national
research and advocacy center working to end hunger and undernutrition
in the United States. Ms. Parker directs FRAC's work on child nutrition
programs, research, and nutrition policy. She played a leadership role in
the development of FRAC's Community Childhood Hunger Identification
Project, a ground-breaking survey of childhood hunger in the United States.
She leads FRAC's initiative on understanding and responding to the para-
dox of hunger, poverty, and obesity. She has authored and edited numerous
publications on hunger, nutrition policy, and federal nutrition programs;
has presented Congressional testimony; and has made speeches and media
appearances on nutrition policy issues that affect low-income communities.
She has served on the Food and Nutrition Board of the Institute of Medicine, on the Technical Advisory Group to America's Second Harvest 2001
and 2005 National Hunger Surveys, on the National Nutrition Monitoring Advisory Council (appointed by then Senate Majority Leader George
Mitchell), and as President of the Society for Nutrition Education. Before
joining FRAC, she worked with New York State's Expanded Food and Nutrition Education Program at Cornell University. Ms. Parker holds a B.A.
in anthropology from the University of Michigan and an M.S. in human
nutrition from Cornell University.

DAVID L. PELLETIER, PH.D., is an Associate Professor of Nutrition
Policy in the Division of Nutritional Sciences at Cornell University, Ithaca,
New York. His teaching and research focuses broadly on strengthening the
methods of policy analysis and development related to food and nutrition.
Dr. Pelletier's research interests include the role of malnutrition in child
mortality, the regulation of dietary supplements and genetically engineered
foods, iron fortification, and methods for participatory planning and policy
analysis at community and national levels. One of his current efforts is
The Whole Community Project, an action research project in upstate New
York designed to examine the prospects and requirements for communities

to succeed in preventing childhood obesity. He has served as a consultant to or member of several international government and nongovernmental organizations including The World Health Organization, Pan American Health Organization, UNICEF, The World Bank, International Food Policy Research Institute, U.S. Agency for International Development, and the Life Sciences Research Office. Dr. Pelletier served on IOM/NRC projects including the Subcommittee on Food and Health for the Opportunities in Agriculture Project, and the International Food and Nutrition Forum. Dr. Pelletier earned a B.A. degree in anthropology and a B.S. degree in biology from the University of Arizona, and M.A. and Ph.D. degrees in anthropology from Pennsylvania State University.

MARY STORY, PH.D., R.D., is a Professor in the Division of Epidemiology and Community Health, School of Public Health, and an Adjunct Professor in the Department of Pediatrics, School of Medicine, at the University of Minnesota, Minneapolis. Dr. Story also serves as Director of Healthy Eating Research, National Program Office, a Robert Wood Johnson Foundation funded initiative. Her Ph.D. is in nutrition and her research focuses on eating behaviors of children and youth and interventions for obesity prevention, with specific focus on low-income and minority communities. Dr. Story received awards from the American Public Health Association, the American Dietetic Association, the Association of State and Territorial Public Health Nutrition Directors, and the Minnesota Department of Health. She is active in national professional associations and is a past chair of the Food and Nutrition Section of the American Public Health Association. Dr. Story served on the IOM Committee on Food Marketing and the Diets of Children and Youth.

Index